Quit or Die

The Truth About Alcohol

Heart Breaking Near-Death Survivor Stories

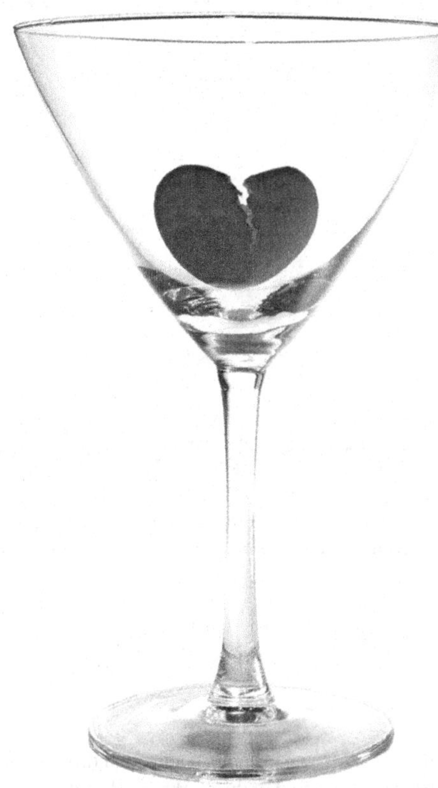

The Solution To The Alcohol Epidemic

Your Key To Success In Sobriety!

How to Sober Up, Quit Drinking,
And Have A Better Life Without Booze

Joy Peters, PhD
Celebrity Anti-Aging Doctor & Addiction Counselor

Order this book online at www.trafford.com
or email orders@trafford.com

Most Trafford titles are also available at major online book retailers.

Print information available on the last page.

ISBN: 978-1-4907-9523-2 (sc)
ISBN: 978-1-4907-9650-5 (e)

Trafford rev. 09/27/2019

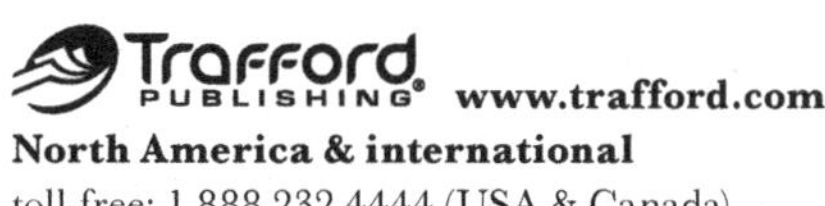

www.trafford.com

North America & international
toll-free: 1 888 232 4444 (USA & Canada)
fax: 812 355 4082

Contents

Foreword

Cheers! To our tee-totaling President Donald Trump. Thanks for being a good example of sobriety for all the American people and thanks for the good business advice that you personally gave me:

> *"Do what you love and love what you do but most importantly, develop Stick-To-It-Tiveness. If you develop Stick-To-It-Tiveness you will be successful in all you do."*

A Quote by President Donald Trump
To The Author

Special Dedication

To all those still fighting their own battle against Alcoholism. I pray that God strengthens your mind, body and spirit to overcome and conquer the forces of alcohol and may you enjoy all the best things that life has to offer, thereafter. May you be blessed with sobriety, good health, peace, love, joy and a long and healthy life and share your success story with others that you can be an inspiration to. Amen!

Special Thanks

To Lillian Peters, the kindest but strongest woman I've ever known, my mom. Thanks for always being a good example to your family on how to be strong and face problems naturally by never drinking or doing drugs and for always encouraging me not to.

To Mikel Ravenscroft. Thanks for being alcohol-free and encouraging me to be. Thanks for inspiring and motivating me. Thanks for being my best friend and for all you do to help others.

To Summer Perry, my daughter. Thanks for being the intelligent person you are to resist alcohol use and for letting go of the past and being your own best example through a natural inner strength and wisdom with a keen sense of making the world a better place than you found it. You are an awe-inspiring and shining example of inner beauty, self-awareness and self-healing.

In Memory of….

Mark Perry 5/29/61-3/3/17
and to all those who fought and died in their battle against alcoholism. R.I.P.

Chapter 1

When you think of having a drink or a cocktail, like many others, you may associate it with relaxing, partying, laughing and having a good time with your friends. It's true, we've all been sold on that happy-go-lucky idea of having fun on alcohol. Every second, someone is raising a glass to toast some special occasion. Alcohol has become a part of almost every celebration in America, holidays, vacations, ball games, birthday parties, concerts, music festivals and even social business events. Most people think they are going to go out and drink a few drinks and have a good time, but many wake up in an Alcohol induced hell filled with ill health, lost relationships, legal problems, DUI's, fines, jail time or job loss and some don't wake up at all, they die. Don't let Alcohol turn your dreams into a nightmare. 86.4 percent of American adults, over 18, reported that they have drank alcohol. All of us have a choice to make about drinking. Either we quit drinking or we decide to drink our whole lives until we die from something related to drinking, it's your choice. This book is designed to help you quit drinking and help you and your loved ones reclaim your health, motivation, energy and joy for life without Alcohol. You can gain control over Alcohol for a better life and future. Alcohol has become so commonly used that we have become desensitized to its dangers.

When people hear about alcohol abuse many may think it is just about the bar scene, college kids getting drunk, teens gone-wild, chugging beer-bongs but alcohol abuse is not restricted to the typical college frat party anymore. In fact, people are doing crazy things with alcohol, now, anything from butt chugging to huffing, inhaling, vaping, smoking it and doing eye-shots! Yes, some are literally, injecting alcohol into their eye-sockets! Why? Because of some false urban legend rumor that you can avoid having the smell of alcohol on your breath and avoid putting on the pounds by these other methods of alcohol consumption because the alcohol is not metabolised through the digestive tract. However, they fail to mention these methods can cause nerve and brain damage and these beliefs are dangerously incorrect and are potentially even more health damaging and deadly than drinking alcohol.

What is Alcohol

The same type of alcohol found in alcoholic beverages is used as fuel. It is ethanol and is most often used as a motor fuel, mainly as a biofuel additive for gasoline. Ethanol fuel is ethyl alcohol. However, if you were to drink gas your kidneys would shut down and you would die, because there are many other additives and petroliate chemicals added to gasoline for combustion engines. Drinking gasoline causes kidney failure, alimentary tract burns and swelling, vision loss, blood stools, blood vomiting, kidney, heart and blood collapse, burning of respiratory track and death. Drinking alcohol causes damage, too.

How Does Alcohol Intoxicate Us?

When we drink an alcoholic beverage, as it is consumed a small amount of alcohol is absorbed sublingually into the bloodstream through the mucous membranes, the majority of it passes through our mouths. down the esophagus and into the stomach. There it is digested into the small intestine and that is where most of the alcohol enters our bloodstream through the walls of the small intestine. Alcohol is a carbohydrate. Alcoholic beverages are mainly carbohydrates with a chemical structure that partially resembles sugar but carbohydrates do not contain ethanol as alcoholic beverages do. During metabolism our bodies burn carbohydrates in alcohol and carbohydrates in the foods we eat in order to gain energy. Burning carbohydrates also produces carbonic acid, which goes into the bloodstream via the small intestine. When this carbonic acid goes through the bloodstream and through the lungs, they remove the acidic part of it through exhalation as carbon dioxide which then leaves only the remaining water in the bloodstream. This removal of carbon dioxide by the lungs is the body's quickest way to reduce blood acidity. The blood from the heart contains a very small amount of carbon dioxide. When we drink alcohol it ignites the metabolism so quickly that the lungs cannot exhale all of the carbon dioxide and part of it reaches the brain and that is when we become intoxicated because this blood brings carbon dioxide to the brain instead of oxygen. The extra calories and carbs we can't exhale or burn off are transmutated to fatty acids that become fatty deposits that accumulate in the body until the liver can produce enough enzymes to break down the fat and eventually turns to fatty liver disease when there is never enough enzymes over a long period of time. The body preferentially oxidizes carbohydrates rather than fat oxidation because it provides more energy and lipids are more energy dense than carbohydrates allowing for more stored energy than can occur in muscle and liver cells. This is how glucose can be converted to fat, leading to weight gain, high cholesterol and fatty liver disease associated with alcohol use.

Seriousness of Alcohol In America

As you already know, Alcohol is not always all fun and games and it has become a serious crisis in America. Millions are suffering from the negative consequences of alcohol. America is in an alcohol crisis. Alcohol is the single most used and abused drug in America and Alcoholism is on the rise but you don't have to be an alcoholic to die from alcohol. Alcohol poisoning kills many who are new to experimenting with alcohol and kills many drinkers, too.

Alcohol Risk Over 50

Recent studies show that it is not only the youth of the nation who are boozing it up. In fact, seniors 50+ are engaging in dangerous levels of alcohol use, as well. Keep in mind Alcohol can complicate the risk of other adult onset illnesses, such as high blood pressure, type II diabetes and high cholesterol. Mid-life and beyond is a time of life where alcohol consumption poses an even greater risk to your health. From mid-life to old age, it is a serious gamble to your health by over drinking alcohol. Getting drunk over 60 is one of the most dangerous health risks for elderly people as falls are a number one cause of hip fractures and death.

Age Groups Most Affected By Alcohol

Alcohol is negatively affecting the quality of life in humans of all ages, prenatal infants to geriatrics, babies to grandparents. Only 30% of the population did not drink last year, that means 70% of the population reported having alcohol and according to a previous 2015 National Survey on Drug Use and Health 86.4 % of people ages 18 or older reported that they drank alcohol at some point in their lifetime and a new study shows that 32 million Americans have struggled with a serious alcohol drinking problem. 13.8 million Americans are alcoholics. Binge drinking is highest among young adults, but deaths from alcohol poisoning within this age group are the lowest, at 5 percent. Young people will stay awake longer and can tolerate higher amounts of alcohol and 3 out of 4 alcohol-poisoning deaths involve adults ages 35 to 64 with the highest deaths among people who are 45 to 54 years old. Widowers over 75 have the highest rate of alcoholism in the United States An astounding 2.5 million older adults have drug or alcohol problems. Seniors may not be the first group to come to mind when you think about alcoholism, but maybe they should be. Alcoholism can develop at any stage in life, but it can be especially damaging to the elderly. It is clear that alcohol is a serious problem that affect many people.

Alcohol and You

If you have an Alcohol problem, your not alone and please, know this, there is hope, there is help and you can kick-the-habit. Alcohol is not all fun and games. Three-fourths of Americans are self-medicating their pain with alcohol and other substances. The misuse of alcohol ruins lives and families. America has a drinking problem, worse than ever before and it's getting worse. We hope that this book helps you and those you love or care for to gain control over alcohol. Now, let's begin your awakening journey that will lead you to solutions to help you solve problem drinking so you can enjoy a longer and healthier life.

We Have Been Conditioned To Think Alcohol Is An Adult Reward Like Giving Candy To A Kid

Ancient Alcohol Origins

Humans have been fermenting alcoholic beverages since before 10,000 B.C. and primative people probably felt the effects of natural fermentation from eating decaying fruits, even before then. As far back as the history of the first people, in the ancient land of Sumer, alcohol use was found in the Sumerian cuneiform tablets, dating back to 2200 BC the specific details of the medicinal role of wine making. Wine is the world's oldest documented human-made medicine. Wine continued to play a major role in medicine until the early 20th century when changing opinions and medical research on alcohol and alcoholism cast doubt on its role as part of a healthy lifestyle. The facts are the negative side effects far outweigh the few positive benefits.

What is Your Poison? What People Are Drinking?

Beer has typically been the preferred alcoholic beverage in the U.S. Gallup poll studies Gallup has also found that beer is more popular among men as 62% of male drinkers say they prefer beer, compared to 19% of female drinkers. However, women account for drinking 57% of wine volume sales in the U.S.

The Top Most Sold Forms of Alcoholic Beverages

#1 - Beer with 62% of total alcohol sales

Spirits/ Hard Liquor - 37% of the sales of all alcohol sales.

Sub-categories:
#2 - Vodka with 34%
#3 - Whiskey with 24%
#4 - Wine 15%
#5 - Rum with 12%

Annual American Alcohol Spendings

According to the National Institutes of Health. In 2017, Americans bought over $72 billion dollars worth of alcohol in the United States. According to the NIH, just that one year of revenue from the people purchases of alcoholic beverages could fund all

NIH-sponsored research on alcoholism, alcohol use and effects of alcohol on health for the next 143 years. Alcohol manufacturing companies are amongst the richest in the nation.

Alcohol Spirits

Alcoholic beverages are distilled producing ethanol by means of fermenting herbs, grains, fruits or vegetables with an alcohol content of 20% and are called spirits. However, many people of religious faith will argue that alcohol is the opposite of holy water and in a sense is a sort of devil water and from that perspective, the reason alcohol is referred to as "spirits" is because it can weaken the body and open up a portal for evil spirits to invade and possess a person.

American Culture Alcohol Use By Ethnicity & Gender

Studies consistently show that Caucasians are consuming more alcohol than other ethnic groups. The biggest binge-drinkers, however, are Hispanics, at 25% closely followed by 24.8 % of Caucasians, 24.1 % of Multi-Racial Americans, 19.8 % of African Americans and 11.1% are Asian Americans. Additionally, women, in general, account for drinking 57% of all wine and women have a higher mortality rate from alcoholism than men.

Men Vrs Women

In the United States, males drink more often and more heavily than females, consuming greater than twice as much alcohol per year equating to 18 liters of pure alcohol for males and 7.8 liters for females according to the NIAAA team in the journal Alcoholism and Clinical and Experimental Research. However, government studies show American women battling alcohol use is growing. Men in every age group prefer beer to wine and liquor. Wine is the preferred drink of women. Beer is the preferred alcoholic beverage of men aged 18 to 49. Men over 50 prefer. Fewer than 1 in 10 male drinkers aged 18 to 29 drink wine. For women, low-risk drinking is defined as no more than 3 drinks on any single day and no more than 7 drinks per week. For men, it is defined as no more than 4 drinks on any single day and no more than 14 drinks per week. About 24 % of alcohol poisoning deaths are women and 76 % of alcohol poisoning deaths occur among men, and nearly 70 % occur among non-hispanic whites and only 6% of alcohol poisoning deaths are other male minorities.

Alcohol American History & Future

In a brief look at the history of U.S. drinking indicates that in 1770, the average colonial Americans consumed about three and a half gallons of alcohol per year that is more than double the modern rate. In the 1800's to the 1920's the U.S. had various stringent laws on alcohol and for a period of 13 years, alcohol was illegal with total prohibition. Many times throughout history, when the society was at risk of becoming an alcoholic nation the government has stepped in to regulate alcohol. With the rate of Alcoholism growing in America, you can expect to see more stringent government measures, better educational public health campaigns and alcohol prevention programs. Recently, there have been a myriad of new psychiatric and mental health diagnostic codes relating to alcohol use disorders. Now, Alcoholism is not only a disease it is a psychiatric disorder. Alcohol has long been a part of American culture, since the country's enception, with the exception of the 13 years of prohibition during a ban on the production, importation, transportation and sale of alcoholic beverages from 1920 to 1933. Today, alcohol is consumed world-wide, except in a few countries where it is still prohibited.

History Alcoholism As A Disease

According to Wikipedia, "Alcoholism is characterized by binge drinking and a slow downward slide into helplessness" In 1849, the Swedish Physician Magnus Huss was the first to systematically classify the damage that was attributable to alcohol ingestion. Huss considered the condition to be a chronic, relapsing disease. Jalane Ki was a Swedish scientist who coined the term alcoholism, he was the physician to Swedish kings. R. Brinkley Smithers, an American philanthropist and founder of the Christopher D. Smithers Foundation, which had been named after his father a founder and a director of IBM he was a self-claimed "recovering alcoholic", he donated a total of more than $90 million dollars throughout his lifetime toward alcohol research and treatment programs, more than $40 million to alcoholism programs; $13.5 million through the Smithers Foundation, and $28 million from his own his personal funds. Jellinek coined the expression "the disease concept of alcoholism" and significantly accelerated the movement towards the medicalization of drunkenness and alcohol habituation. Jellinek's initial 1946 study was funded by Marty Mann and R. Brinkley Smithers. It was based on a narrow, selective study of a hand-picked group of members of Alcoholics Anonymous (AA) who had returned a self-reporting questionnaire.

Why Do People Like Alcohol & Why It Is A Health Risk

Alcohol initially stimulates feel good Neurotransmitters (NTs) in the brain. Genetic characteristics may predispose individuals to be more or less susceptible to becoming addicted to alcohol. Over time an alcohol drinker loses substantial control over their voluntary behavior and at some point it becomes compulsive. For many people these behaviors are truly uncontrollable after alcohol dependency has developed. Neurotransmitters are chemicals stimulated by amino-acids, peptides and neuropeptides and are produced by various glands including the pineal gland, pituitary gland and hypothalamus. Alcohol may mimic neurotransmitters. Neurotransmitters communicate information in our brain to regulate our bodily functions. They send signals between nerves via "neurons." There are two types of neurotransmitters:

- **Inhibitory:** serotonin which relaxes, calms and feelings of well-being
- **Excitatory:** epinephrine which stimulates motivation, energy and action

Neurotransmitters regulate mood, sleep, mental concentration, appetite, weight, heart rate and they even signal your lungs to breathe and your stomach to digest. They can also cause adverse symptoms when they are out of balance. Neurotransmitter levels can be depleted from drinking alcohol on a regular basis. As a matter of fact, it is estimated that 86% of Americans have suboptimal neurotransmitter levels because stress, smoking, alcohol, caffeine and a poor diet. Additionally, neurotoxins, genetics, drugs (prescription or recreational) all can cause NT levels to be imbalanced and dysfunctional that is when alcohol doesn't feel good and begins to destroy health. Genes do not doom a person to become an addict but can make some people more prone to addiction and compulsive behaviors.

Alcohol The 1st Medicine

Alcohol has a long and misleading history from being touted as an early form of medication. Wine was once upon a time, commonly recommended as a safe alternative to drinking water! Beer was originally brewed as a kidney remedy to flush out stones. Whiskey was used as a pain reliever for dental and surgical procedures. Gin was originally brewed as a child bearing medicine and health tonic. The mood altering content of Wine is alcohol. If it was used in a medicinal dose it would be considered an ancient medicine, however, in modern society it is used to get drunk. Getting drunk is a health deterrent and health risk. In ancient medicine, alcohol was used as a topical antiseptic for treating wounds, and wine was used as a digestive aid to calm a nervous stomach. Wine was pushed by early chemist and doctors, as a cure for a wide range of ailments including lethargy, diarrhea and pain from childbirth. However, many studies have found no such healthy effects of regular drinking of alcohol and drinking more than a small amount increases the risk of heart disease, high blood pressure, atrial fibrillation, stroke and cancer which proves alcohol is more counter productive to good health and there are no safe levels of regular consumption. In retrospect, no more than a swig of whiskey or wine for was used for pain, in the days before anesthesia, and if it was truly an organically grown grape and no more than a 1 oz. portion size of wine, or a tablespoon of other spirits, such as in cough syrup would be beneficial. Currently, any other use for medicinal reasons is considered barbaric medicine!

Sobering Facts About Alcohol

Alcohol researchers have said having a glass of wine a day is good for us, other studies say that it is bad and does more damage than good. Regardless, alcohol is a drug, alcohol is addictive and alcohol damages your organs, liver and brain, in particular. Even a glass of wine a day does more harm than good. Alcohol increases risk of all kinds of cancers. Acetaldehyde sticks to our DNA that can cause damaged cells then can cause damaged cells to mutate into cancer. 6% of cancers are caused by alcohol in the U.S. Drinking only 5 drinks per week increases your risk of cancer to 13%. Everyone's risk of cancer increases with just one glass a day, regardless if it improves cardiovascular risk it increases your risk of getting cancer.

Alcohol Is A Drug

Dissociatives are a class of hallucinogens which distort perceptions of sight and sound and produce feelings of detachment and dissociation from the environment and one's own self. Some drugs, such as Ketamine are dissociative drugs which have been used as a "date rape" drug because they have a strong dissociative effect and dream-like states or trances which other drugs, such as alcohol and cannabis may cause dissociation in some people but not in others which largely depends on the ingested amount and type of alcohol. The indica strain of cannabis is more of a dissociative and the sativa strain is not likely a dissociative.

Toxins In Wine

Obviously, the first issue with wine as the first medicine, is that it contains alcohol. Wine Is Not Anti-Aging Potion. Ethanol oxidized to ethanoic acid in wine. Yes, wine is filled with antioxidants, but the alcohol content of the wine is more negative than the positive benefit of thc antioxidant. Wine would have been a beneficial medicine in a teaspoon sized dose as the Sumerians intended, if it were only made of organic grapes, sugar, yeast and water, but it is not. Wine is often full of toxins from growing and processing from field to bottle. Too much of a good thing, is a bad thing. A culture of over-indulgence has taken wine and turned it into a health robbing villain. First of all, the juice of any fruit should never be consumed in an amount of over 1 oz in a 24 hour period, as without the fiber in the fruit juice spikes blood sugar and fruit juices have a high glycemic index which stresses the pancreas and causes blood sugar problems and which may lead to diabetes and obesity, when over consumed. Drinking dry wine actually causes your blood sugar to drop because your body focuses on metabolizing the alcohol calories first before food calories. In 2008, researchers from Kingston University in London discovered the second worst problem with drinking too much red wine, as it contains high levels of toxic metals relative to other beverages in the sample. In an investigation of wine production, sulfites triggers asthma and allergies, it can cause negative side effects, like nasal congestion, itchy throat, a runny nose, skin rash, and hives in some people. Exposure to sulfites is a common cause of excessive inflammation and pain. 5% of people have a strong allergic reaction to sulfites. including the influence that grape variety, soil type, geographical region, insecticides, containment in fermenting vessels and seasonal variations may be a culprit in the toxic metal ion uptake in grape crops, juice processing and wine fermentation processes and procedures. Additionally, the third worst issue with wine is there are preservatives, sulfites and flavor enhancers in wine that can have an accumulative adverse effect on human health as it is metabolized in the body. What may be safe legal amounts of chemicals, per serving, by manufacturing standards, may not be a safe level in the body of an alcohol abuser who over consumes, in excess of a single serving and therefore the chemical residues would be considered a toxic level risk that can be cumulative in the body.

Religion and Wine

Sacramental wine, communion wine, or altar wine is wine obtained from grapes and intended for use in celebration of the Eucharist, Lord's Supper or Holy Communion. It is usually consumed after sacramental bread, although historically the wine was reserved for clergy. Again, the wine is taken in a sip, not in a five ounce serving size that is typical, today. The Bible also gives many references and stern warnings against being drunk. Ephesians 5:18: Do not be drunk with wine. Some studies show that those of faith who use wine as sacrament are more prone to abuse wine in their personal lives, as well. In fact, Vatican City, consumes more wine, per capita, than any other place on the planet. In the Vatican city, the average resident consumes 52.6 liters of wine, annually. Why would religion utilize so much wine? It's in the bible, however many biblical scholars insist the wine in the bible was unfermented wine. In the Hebrew Bible, Noah planted a vineyard and became inebriated. Drunkenness is discouraged in the bible and some biblical persons abstained from alcohol. In the bible, Alcohol is used symbolically, in both positive and negative terms. Its consumption is prescribed for religious rites or medicinal uses. In the new testament, Jesus miraculously turned water to wine. Wine is the most common alcoholic beverage mentioned in the bible as it is a source of symbolism and was a part of daily life. According to the bible, in ancient Israel they drank beer and wines made from other fruits. Since alcohol abuse, is progressive and can develop into alcoholism, it is best for your health to heed biblical warnings which is as valid, from a religious stance, than consuming alcohol as sacrament.

Chapter 2

Geographics Of Alcohol Use - U.S. vs Other Countries

Not only is Alcohol a problem in the United States, it is a problem on a global level. The U.S. ranks number 3 in the list of countries with the most drug and alcohol dependencies by population. Americans are only 5% of the world's population and yet, Americans consume more than 80% of the narcotic pharmaceuticals manufactured. Those who consume other drugs are at a high risk of serious and life threatening complications by combining drugs with Alcohol. Culture has a huge bearing in the use of the type of alcohol used in various countries. Ironically, Catholics are the top wine consumers in the world. The regions which Catholics live rank amongst the highest wine consumption in the world. In India, an alcoholic beverage called sura, distilled from rice, was in use between 3000 and 2000 B.C. but now some regions of India it is prohibited. The Babylonians worshiped a wine goddess as early as 2700 B.C. In Greece, one of the first alcoholic beverages to gain popularity was mead, a fermented drink made from honey and water.

There is a culture influence on every form of alcohol consumed. Southerners are more inclined to drink beer, just as the Irish are more inclined to drink whiskey, and Russia drinks the most vodka. Basically, the variety of alcohol consumption relates to what the region produces most and the crops that are readily available for the production of alcohol products.

Regardless, of global difference, one thing is in common, everywhere, Alcohol abuse, is progressive and no culture is immune to alcoholism and the negative effects of alcohol are consistent on human health in all cultures .

Drunk Shopping

Not only are Americans spending a fortune on alcohol, a recent survey of alcohol-consuming American adults found that drunk shopping is an estimated $45 billion per year industry and 79% of all drinkers made online purchases while under the influence of alcohol. Drinkers have reported shopping and buying things during an alcoholic blackout that they didn't remember buying until the surprise package arrived and report they would have never bought when they were sober. People drunk shop for sexy clothes, that won't fit over their beer belly and often they wouldn't be caught dead wearing whilst sober. Drunk shoppers often buy things a sober person wouldn't buy, gaudy flashing yard signs and even ridiculous animal costumes for pets.

Population Statistics and Generational Alcohol Consumption

The current population of the United States of America is 328,468,836 (328.5 million) as of Tuesday, March 26, 2019, based on the latest United Nations estimates. The median age in the United States is 37.8 years. Millennials are the majority of the American population, now. There are 84 million millennials. Millennials are citizens between the age of 22ish to 35ish. Millenials make up 26 % of the total population they are not only the largest living generation today but also millennials are the majority workforce, they make up 75 % of the American workforce. Millennials drank around 159.6 million cases of wine last year, an amount that surpasses any other generation. Millennials drank 42% of all wine consumed in 2015 and the new study estimates are projected to be even higher.

We Have Been Conditioned To Toast Every Celebration With Alcohol

Many millenials are consuming alcohol in quantities above the maximum recommended serving for men and women on a daily basis, the average millenial drinker consumes around 3.1 glasses a sitting according to a report by the Wine Market Council. Additionally, women, in general, account for drinking 57% of all wine. Millenials are known as the wellness-generation, with all their fitness clothing, wellness gadgets and wearable fitness technology, but in comparison with other generations, the wine drinking habits of millennials are even more alarming than ever before. Additionally, many of the millenial's grand-parents, the baby boomers, guzzled 30% of all wine consumed in the U.S. while Millennial parents, Generation X, sipped down only 20% of the wine. 17% of all millennial wine drinkers bought a bottle costing over $20 in the past month, compared to 10% of all drinkers and compared to only 5% of Baby Boomers who are consuming more beer.

Alcohol is an Obstacle to be Eliminated On Your Path To Achieving An Optimal Life Experience.

It appears that, even though Millenials are considered the wellness generation they are the largest generation of heavy wine drinkers. Millennials tend to be more frugal and health conscious than prior generations, but they do have a great deal of stress, trying to clean up the many messes previous generations left for them to deal including global warming, cleaning up the oceans. It is possible that many millenials, could be self-medicating with the enormous amounts of the wine they are consuming. Are millenials trying to drink away their problems? How are they coping with the frustrations of stricter rules imposed upon them from the mistakes of previous generations resulting in the forced obligation of carrying the burden of the enormous national debt, global warming and other problems left behind for them to resolve and pay for.

Millennial Health Oxymorons

Millenials are the most wellness focused population group yet have more stress as a factor leading to self-medicating with alcohol. Millennials stress over securing desirable jobs and assuming the high baby boomer, national debt to be paid off by their generation. Just as the economy is getting over the 2008 housing bubble nightmare that their boomer parents also helped create, now Millennials must deal with the impending 2019 housing bubble causing many millenials to be unable to easily acquire bank loans from home lenders without huge down payments and perfect credit scores, which high student loan debts affect and other financial difficulties. Many are dealing with personal frustrations of not being able to afford their first homes because they suffer the consequences of the stringent post housing bubble bank lending rules. Also, the economy is still shaky and recovering from the stock market collapse. The new 2019 housing bubble is making financing the average millennial first home purchases difficult to near impossible, for most. All of these stress factors can increase the tendency to self-medicate and imposes a higher risk of substance abuse in the millennial demographic. These are only some of the reasons, the millenials are a high risk group for addiction and alcoholism. Many millennials are super intelligent techie types others are strong problem solvers and millennials have a passion to make the world a better place than it is. Millenials are young and there is still time to change the course of the future, hopefully, the millennials will not allow alcohol to become their demise.

Millennial Alcohol Deaths

It is shocking that young millennial aged adults are seeing greater increases in liver disease deaths than any other age group. Numbers are rising in both the number of deaths from liver disease and the number of those who have died from alcohol-related cirrhosis. Cirrhosis is the latest stage of liver damage. Alcohol-related liver disease deaths among millennials increased 10% each year since the recession, according to the study. Deaths from liver disease have increased sharply in recent years in the United States, according to a study published in the British Medical Journal. Cirrhosis-related deaths increased by 65 % from 1999 to 2016, and deaths from liver cancer doubled, the study concluded.

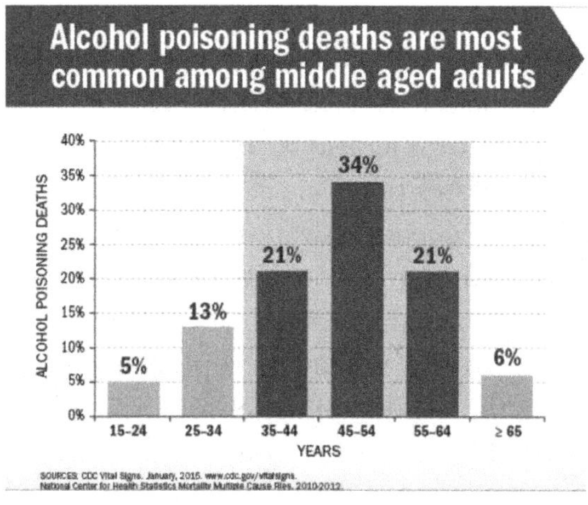

Baby Boomer Death By Alcohol Risk

Alcohol-related deaths have increased dramatically in Baby Boomers. The number of alcohol-specific deaths in people aged 50 and over has risen 45%. There were 5,208 deaths in people over 50 that were directly caused by alcohol, last year. Quitting will prove difficult due to the Baby-Boomer lifestyle that involves regular drinking of alcohol but it is never too late to quit drinking. Baby Boomers are the generation with the highest risk of dying from an alcohol related death.

Baby Boomer Vs Millennial - Majority Alcoholism

The Baby Boomers and Millennials are the two largest generational populations in America. The Baby boomers grew up in an age when there was less information about the dangers of alcohol. Baby Boomers represents 33% of America's population, while consuming 45% of the nation's alcohol.

It Is Never Too Late To Quit

Alcohol has done much damage to Baby Boomers health and many have already died of alcohol related problems and for many more baby boomers it is almost too late as baby boomer deaths surge from lifetime of alcohol abuse. Millennials still have time on their side, to change their future health destiny and can dodge the bullet of alcoholism by quitting alcohol now and focusing on a wellness lifestyle, better physical and mental health and become a healthier generation instead of repeating the failures of past generations. Millennials are the Mocktail generation.

American Minorities And Alcohol Use

According to the U.S. Department of Health and Human Services and the National Institutes of Health in an Alcohol Alert dated March 2002, In respect to the four main minority groups of United States citizens: African Americans; Hispanic Americans; Asian Americans and Pacific Islanders and American Indians/Alaska Natives. People vary in their vulnerability to the effects of alcohol. Some of these differences result from genetically determined variations in the body's ability to break down and eliminate alcohol. For example, after drinking, many Asian subpopulations experience flushing of the skin, nausea, headache, and other uncomfortable symptoms. Those symptoms result primarily from inactivity of aldehyde dehydrogenase ($ALDH_2$), an enzyme involved in a key step of alcohol metabolism. A study of Asian males born in Canada and the United States found that those who had inherited the gene for the less active form of this enzyme drank two-thirds less alcohol, had one-third the rate of binge drinking, and were three times more likely to be abstainers than a group of Asian males who possessed the more active enzyme. However, some people develop alcohol problems despite possessing the inactive form of ALDH2, demonstrating the importance of additional factors in the development of drinking patterns and consequences. Among some African Americans, genetically determined variability in another alcohol-metabolizing enzyme, alcohol dehydrogenase-2, appears to affect the degree of vulnerability to alcoholic cirrhosis and alcohol-related fetal damage.

Jobs With Highest Alcohol Death Rates

According to a database of 11 million death certificates sorted by cause of death and occupation compiled by the National Institute for Occupational Safety and Health revealed the following alcoholism deaths by profession.

The following professions are more likely to die from alcoholism than average

1) Bartenders are 2.33 times
2) Shoe machine operators are 2.00 times
3) Roofers are 1.87 times
4) Painters are 1.85 times
5) Cooks are 1.77 times
6) Sailors are 1.75 times
7) Construction laborers are 1.72 times
8) Drywall installers are 1.71 times
9) Musicians are 1.65 times
10) Concrete finishers are 1.65 times
11) Amusement park attendants are 1.61 times
12) Farmers are 1.59 times
13) Surveyors are 1.51 times

Those are the professions more likely to die from alcoholism than average

The Drunkest City In Your State

According to a Centers for Disease Control report, these are the cities in each state with the highest consumption of alcoholic beverages. Living there adds an additional environmental influence increasing the odds of you abusing alcohol and becoming an alcoholic.

1. Alabama: Auburn
2. Alaska: Fairbanks
3. Arizona: Flagstaff
4. Arkansas: Fayetteville-Springdale-Rogers

5. California: Chico
6. Colorado: Fort Collins
7. Connecticut: Bridgeport-Stamford-Norwalk
8. Delaware: Dover
9. Florida: Crestview-Fort Walton Beach-Destin
10. Georgia: Athens-Clarke County
11. Hawaii: Kahului-Wailuku-Lahaina
12. Idaho: Coeur d'Alene
13. Illinois: Bloomington
14. Indiana: Bloomington
15. Iowa: Iowa City
16. Kansas: Lawrence
17. Kentucky: Louisville/Jefferson County
18. Louisiana: Houma-Thibodaux
19. Maine: Portland-South Portland
20. Maryland: California-Lexington Park
21. Massachusetts: Barnstable Town
22. Michigan: Lansing-East Lansing
23. Minnesota: Mankato-North Mankato
24. Mississippi: Gulfport-Biloxi-Pascagoula
25. Missouri: Columbia
26. Montana: Missoula
27. Nebraska: Lincoln
28. Nevada: Reno
29. New Hampshire: Manchester-Nashua
30. New Jersey: Ocean City
31. New Mexico: Santa Fe
32. New York: Watertown-Fort Drum
33. North Carolina: Jacksonville
34. North Dakota: Fargo
35. Ohio: Columbus
36. Oklahoma: Lawton
37. Oregon: Portland-Vancouver-Hillsboro
38. Pennsylvania: State College
39. Rhode Island: Providence-Warwick
40. South Carolina: Hilton Head Island area
41. South Dakota: Sioux Falls
42. Tennessee: Nashville area
43. Texas: Austin-Round Rock
44. Utah: Salt Lake City
45. Vermont: Burlington-South Burlington
46. Virginia: Blacksburg-Christiansburg-Radford
47. Washington: Seattle-Tacoma-Bellevue

48. West Virginia: Morgantown
49. Wisconsin: Green Bay
50. Wyoming: Casper
51. Washington, D.C. (highest rate above all cities)

States With Most Alcohol Purchases

Washington D.C. purchases more alcohol per capita than any state except it's not a state, it is a district. New Hampshire, drinks almost double the national average, according to statistics from the Centers for Disease Control and Prevention (CDC) It is thought to be due to high stress in high stakes politics.

10. South Dakota (2.87 gallons per capita)
9. Idaho (2.92 gallons per capita)
8. Alaska (2.94 gallons per capita)
7. Wisconsin (2.98 gallons per capita)
6. Vermont (3.08 gallons per capita)
5. Montana (3.11 gallons per capita)
4. North Dakota (3.26 gallons per capita)
3. Nevada (3.46 gallons per capita)
2. Delaware (3.72 gallons per capita)
1. New Hampshire (4.76 gallons per capita)

The States With Highest Rates Of Alcoholism

The most recent data from the CDC, U.S. Census Poll Studies and the National Institute for Alcohol Abuse to identify the following states reporting the highest levels of adults who binge drink or drink heavily.

1. North Dakota (24.7 percent)
2. Wisconsin (24.5 percent)
3. Alaska (22.1 percent)
4. Montana (21.8 percent)
5. Illinois (21.2 percent)
6. Minnesota (21.1 percent)
7. Iowa (21 percent)
8. Hawaii (20.5 percent)
9. Nebraska (20.4 percent)
10. Michigan (20 percent)

Alcohol and Alcoholism Treatment

America has the greatest physical health care system in the world and a highly efficient mental health system however everyone overlooks emotional health emotional wounds are not something you can just put a Band-Aid on them many people self medicate their emotional wounds with alcohol

Alcohol is a legal substance for all those over the age of 21 that is addictive and can progress into the disease of alcoholism. Alcohol has been made into some legend of passage into adulthood that many feel they must experience. Alcohol blocks more Neurotransmitters and neural pathways than cocaine or heroin yet it is still legal. To quit drinking you must go on an inner journey of emotional awakening! If alcohol has become a problem in your life, it is most important to discover why you drink and confront your destructive shadow-self so you can overcome alcohol use and take control of your life back from alcohol. It is also important, to understand the causes and potential cures. Although some treatment programs believe alcoholism is considered a disease which there is no cure for if you have an early alcohol habit there are several effective professional approaches and there are many self-help measures you can integrate into your sobriety lifestyle. There is a solutions to help you successfully kick the habit of alcohol dependence while learning to love yourself more and living a better life in sobriety. Unlike alcohol programs of the past, there are new treatments, therapies and exercises to help you reclaim your joy in life over alcohol. There are ways to return to a place of self love and joy in life without alcohol.

- Alcohol Addiction- a brain disease where one has a compulsion to drink without the ability to stop and is marked by compulsive behavior.
- Developing, Surviving and Recovering from Addiction depends on many factors.

There is an epidemic of alcoholism and a flash mob alcoholic deaths happen everyday. It is like many are under a hypnotic magic spell, as everybody knows the dangers yet, so many are hooked on this poison we call alcohol.There are hidden culprits of alcoholism, and usually pain and emotional traumas are a factor, as well.

U.S. & Global Alcohol Use & Prohibition

The U.S. consist of people from all over the world. Each ethnic group metabolises alcohol differently and metabolism varies all the way down to each individual. Caucasians have the highest rate of alcohol consumption amongst U.S. citizens but over the past decade, Hispanic drinkers went up 51.9 % and African American alcohol consumption has increased by 92.8 %. The 2007 CIA World Factbook list the religion of France as 83-88% Roman Catholic and Catholic countries drink the most wine. Japan has the longest life expectancy and consumes a liter less of alcohol per capita indicating that longevity goes up as alcohol consumption numbers go down but with France the ratio appear to contradict these statistics. Perhaps the French can metabolise alcohol more efficiently. France has always been keen on portion control, as well. Portion size offsets the general statistics with more strict moderation in food consumption. Not over drinking the portion size can improve longevity and offset the adverse effects of alcohol consumption. France typically has a lower obesity rate and the co-morbidities of obesity compounds the negative effects of alcohol.

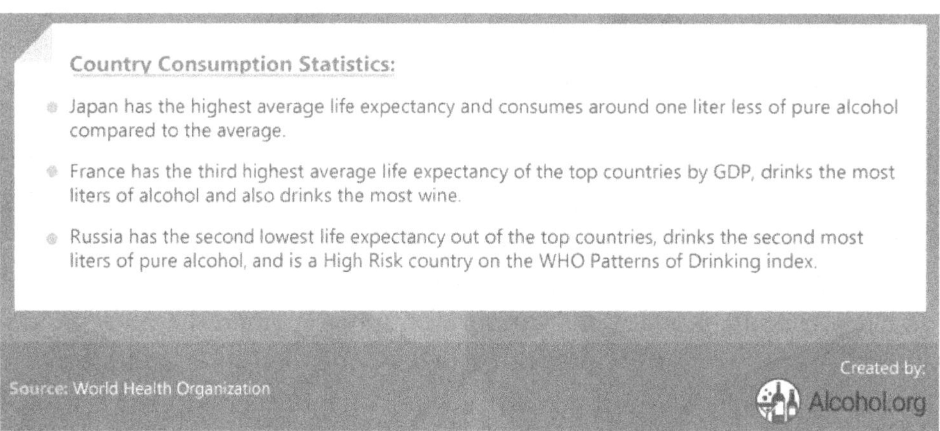

Foreign Culture Influence In American Statistics & The Alcohol Epidemic

Not only is alcohol illegal in some countries due to religious reason but the people from these cultures that live in the U.S. These foreigners are probably improving the actual alcohol stat numbers in our society. Countries ban alcohol because of scientific research of the adverse effects of alcohol as well as the behavior of individuals under its use affects the reasoning within each countries decision to pass an alcohol prohibition act. The goal of these countries is not to control its citizens but protect them.

There are still a few countries where alcohol is prohibited as follows:

- Afghanistan
- Bangladesh
- Brunei
- India (certain states and union territories)
- Iran
- Kuwait
- Libya
- Pakistan (for Muslims
- Saudi Arabia
- Sudan
- United Arab Emirates (in Sharjah)
- Yemen
- Pakistan (for Muslims)

The possession of alcohol in these countries is a crime. Consumption of alcohol in these countries will land the offender in jail. In Pakistan, they still whip people for possession of alcohol crimes and the jail sentence is 3 years and 30 strikes with a whip. What if everytime you bought alcohol meant you were going to be beaten, if you get caught with it, can you imagine? Still we beat our own bodies up every time we drink alcohol. The negative health effects is not just about being inebriated by alcohol it is also, the added toxins in alcohol that are a detriment to your good health.

The Name Alcohol Origination

"Al-kuhl" is Arabic word meaning: body eating spirit. The root origin for the word hol is the English term "ghoul". In folklore, a ghoul is a demon spirit thought to eat human bodies. Some bible teachings say there are demons and evil spirits all around us waiting for an opportunity to get inside and possess the human soul. Alcohol is a tool that causes a person to let down their inhibitions. Additional meanings in ancient arabic mythology as follows:

- Alkol-jeannie or spirit supernatural shape-shifter
- Algol- the head of Medusa will turn onlookers to stone
- Fixed star in astrology which means demons head
- Algol- fixed star in astrology
- Algal- Meaning spirit or demon
- Ghoul- one who shows morbid interest in things considered shocking or repulsive.
- Khol- takes away the mind or covers it

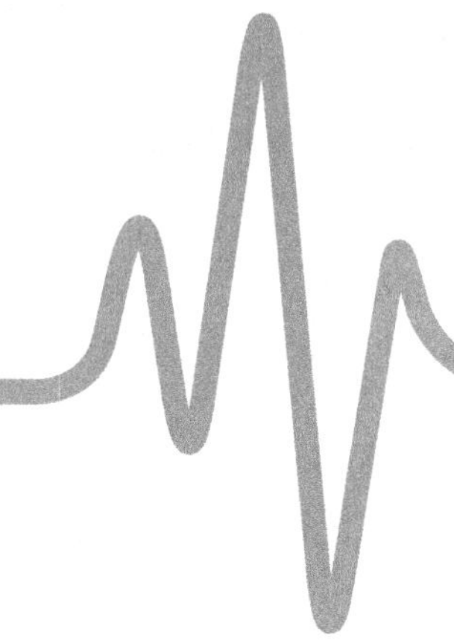

Chapter 3

Toxins in Beer

Many beers contain toxins and the worst allergens, such as lactose, corn, peanut, wheat/gluten and yellow or red food dye, which are carcinogens. Aside from the toxic effects of the alcohol content in beer, the following are some of the not-so-healthy ingredients in beer" and they are also somewhat damaging to your health:

- All kinds of endocrine disruptors linked to hormonal imbalances
- GMO corn, rice, and sugars
- Monosodium Glutamate (MSG)
- Propylene Glycol
- Calcium Disodium EDTA
- Natural Flavors (which aren't natural or healthy)
- High Fructose Corn Syrup
- Caramel Coloring
- Insect-based dyes, and
- Artificial food dyes: FD&C Blue 1, FD&C Red 40, FD&C Yellow 5
- Glyceryl monostearate and pepsin (used for foam
- Carrageenan

Additionally, depending on what type of container beer comes in a drinker may also be getting a dose of toxic metal, aluminum or BPA (a cancer causing plastic), leaching into your beer all of which may affect your physical, mental, emotional and brain health. Lastly, the most cited medical journal, the Lancet published a couple of research studies that show for every extra alcoholic drink over the daily recommended limit, takes ½ hour off your lifespan. Therefore, there are five 12 oz beers in a 60 ounces pitcher of beer. The maximum daily serving for a male is 2 beers, for a woman, only 1 beer. Therefore, if your a guy drinking the whole picture of beer it shortens your lifespan by 1.5 years and for a woman it robs you of 2 years off your life, not to mention stealing your beauty from you. Is it worth it?

Chugging A Picture Of Beer = 2 Years Off Your Life

Toxins in Hard Liquor

Besides the alcohol, some of the toxic ingredients in hard liquor come from chemicals used in how the grain or fruit is grown and processed into ethanol and how it is preserved for bottling. For example, propylene glycol (PG) is found in some whiskey products, it helps prevent sediments forming in liquids during shelf life and it keep liquids from separating but over consumption of propylene glycol or poisoning from it causes primarily central nervous system depression and lactic acidosis. With repeat exposure, PG accumulates in human tissues over time. Other effects on humans include skin and soft tissue necrosis, cardiac dysrhythmias, hypotension, seizure, and hemolysis. According to the National Institutes for Health (NIH), Propylene glycol is primarily metabolized by alcohol dehydrogenase in liver into lactic acid, then pyruvic acid. Propylene glycol is toxic at elevated amounts, which can lead to severe lactic acidosis and renal failure. Also, there are toxins in mixed cocktails as there are many toxins used in the production of the mixers. If you're mixing tequila with margarita mixer, the mixer is more toxic than the tequila or if you mix vodka with raspberry cosmopolitan mixer, artificial flavoring and coloring is full of chemicals that have an accumulative toxic effect, compounded by alcohol when over consumed. Even those going more natural with vodka orange juice, how the fruit was grown can leach toxic farming chemical residues and additionally, if the juice is from concentrate it may contain high fructose GMO grain corn syrup, there really is poison in your poison. A variety of booze is made from grains or fruits that may have been commercially grown, from GMO seeds or may have been sprayed with herbicides and pesticides. You can best avoid potential toxins, allergens and GMOs by abstaining and by leaving hard liquor alone. Remember, corn is a huge GMO crops and even some vodka is now made from corn or grains instead of potatoes. The hidden factors are good reasons to QUIT alcohol.

Alcohol & Aging

Alcohol is dehydrating to the body. Dehydration is your skins worst enemy. Alcohol dilates blood vessels causing collapsing of tiny blood vessels and red blotchy skin. Alcohol is one of the most acidifying substance humans consume, changing the body chemistry and speeding up the aging process. Alcohol accelerates the development of wrinkles and leads to premature aging. Alcohol consumption also contributes to fragile, thinining, frizzy hair and hair loss. The first effect of alcohol accelerated aging is dehydration. In order to metabolize the acidic alcohol, the body will compensate by actually robbing the fluid out of your skin. If you look at a woman who has been drinking for 20 years, and a woman of the same age who hasn't at all, you can see a massive difference in the quality of skin, the drinker has more wrinkles from dehydration damage, and the drinker look 10 years older in appearance.

Alcohol Shortens Life Expectancy

Drinking will shorten your life, according to a study that suggests every extra glass of wine or a pint of beer over the daily recommended limit will cut half an hour from the expected lifespan of a 40-year-old. Alcohol contains sugar which can and does lead to weight gain and obesity and other adult onset illnesses. Lastly, alcohol may cause cancer.

Alcohol Shortens Your Life 1/2 Hour For Every Extra Glass

Homeostasis And Alcohol

Homeostasis is the state of steady internal physical and chemical balance within the body. Homeostasis is the optimal balance and functioning of the innate intelligence of the body's self-healing mechanism. a state of stable equilibrium between interdependent elements in the body. Homeostasis is especially important as it maintains normal functioning of physiological processes. Balance is the key to an optimally functioning nervous system. Examples of homeostasis, is how the body maintains a normal blood pressure or body temperature by homeostasis. The same way the body regulates biochemical homeostasis in the body, the brain keeps balance of brain chemistry with GABA and glutamate. Glutamate is the main excitatory and GABA the main inhibitory neurotransmitter in the human brain cortex. As the two primary inhibitory and excitatory neurotransmitters in the brain and the two perform a balancing act in regulating the central nervous system and our state of excitement or our state of calmness and play a role in the balance of all mental states in between excitement and calmness. Alcohol gradually disrupts homeostasis and though many side effects can be improved with sobriety, alcohol can cause permanent damage in the body.

Chemistry Imbalance And Alcohol

Alcohol use creates imbalances in the body and depletes the body of minerals, electrolytes and in many ways and colloidal minerals supplement the balance of the body's natural chemical production. Colloidal minerals help balance body chemistry however the science is relatively young and the number of qualified experts who are trained to monitor these levels in the body are few compared to other areas of science. Mineral colloid compounds are time-tested in health renewing benefits. Most colloidal mineral formulas contain approximately 70 of the 94 naturally occurring elements, including all of the essential minerals, in trace amounts. Trace minerals are so important that the lack of trace minerals quite possibly may be one of the primary causes of illness in the western culture diet, today. It has been scientifically proven that these vital colloidal minerals are insufficient in the standard food diet that americans typically eat and adding alcohol to the mix robs the bones of calcium buffers and therefore mineral supplementation must be added to our diet for balance, optimal health and longevity. Some of the possible benefits of supplementing with plant-source trace minerals are:

- Balances ph
- aids absorption of vitamins
- Replenishes diminished nutrient reserves
- provides general chemistry balance
- helps to build and maintain a healthier body
- can increase the flow of energy

Individually, trace minerals have been found to be beneficial for a number of health needs, such as:

- building bones and muscle tissue, stimulating the nervous system, also essential for the proper utilization of calcium *(boron)*
- regulating the breakdown of sugar and carbohydrates *(chromium)*
- helps form red blood cells and maintain nerve tissue *(cobalt)*
- strengthening bones and teeth *(fluoride)*
- regulating the thyroid *(iodine)*
- stimulates a healthy immune system *(iron)*
- fighting cancer cells *(manganese)*
- essential for protein synthesis and nervous system *(molybdenum)*
- destroys free radicals with vitamin E *(selenium)*
- Enzyme precursor and antibiotic capabilities *(sulfur)*
- helping wounds heal, production of white blood cells *(zinc)*

How Advanced Is Your Alcohol Use or Addiction? A Quizz

Please, answer yes or no to the following questions:

1. They think your weak because you can't control your drinking
2. You tell people your are reducing your drinking but you don't.
3. They wonder and ask you why you just can't quit.
4. You feel immense guilt when you wake up the morning after.
5. Guilt trip is painful because your failing in some aspect of life.
6. They Threaten To Leave You
7. They keep you in line by nagging you about your drinking
8. They Say, Just Stop But You Can't
9. They Say, Have Some Discipline, but you can't
10. People are insensitive to you having an alcohol habit .
11. People don't understand why you can't quit?
12. You say, it's not that you can't quit, it's just that you won't quit
13. You can't just say no when it comes to alcohol

14. You love drinking, though you know it's wrecking your life
15. You know the odds of getting cancer from alcohol are high
16. You think you are one of the people who has the genetics
17. One of your parents drank or was an alcoholic
18. Traditional treatment failed to help you
19. They say they are disappointed in you
20. You are unable to drink in moderation
21. You won't stop until the bottle is empty
22. You went through a 12-step program and it didn't work for you.
23. You can't imagine not drinking again for the rest of your life
24. You plan to drink again
25. It is uncomfortable not to have a drink when you want one

If you answered yes to 3, it is likely that you have an alcohol abuse problem. If you answered yes to 6 or more, you are at risk for alcohol addiction. If you answered yes to 9 or more, you are on your way to alcoholism. If you answered yes to 12 or more, you are already an alcoholic.

Who Is Struggling With Alcohol?

18 million people struggle with alcohol addiction in the world, everyday. You are not alone. Even other mammals get addicted to alcohol, monkeys eat fermented fruit and rats will binge drink on alcohol in research labs. It is not a moral failing It is not because your a bad person. Yes, you made the unwise decision to drink to the point of addiction. Alcohol abuse kills more people than 3 million people each year, globally.The craving for alcohol by anyone who is addicted to alcohol is agonizing.

Alcohol addiction is real and the cravings are worse than those experienced with crack or heroin

Alcohol Causes Chemically Induced Neurotransmitter Deficiency

Drinking Alcohol becomes addictive because the alcohol interrupts the production of neuropeptides and neurotransmitters and then the brain gets used to the alcohol as a replacement and becomes dependant in order to function but it doesn't function as properly as it does with the real neurotransmitters. Alcohol hijacks the neural pathways and one of the ways the neurotransmitters and endorphins are released after drinking alcohol is because it acts as an artificial reward system in the brain. In addition, research indicates genetic factors also influence alcohol addiction. Additionally, acetaldehyde released into the brain via catalase metabolism can combine with neurotransmitters to form tetrahydroisoquinolines and some scientists think they are the cause of alcoholism.

Regardless, alcohol interferes with the reuptake of serotonin this is why some drinkers become aggressive. Alcohol replaces the production of "feel good" neurotransmitters and that is another factor in the development of alcohol dependence and withdrawal while quitting alcohol. Neuropeptides, neurotransmitters, growth factors, epinephrine, serotonin, acetylcholine and gamma-aminobutyric acid (GABA) are produced in the pituitary gland of the brain.

Alcohol affects homeostasis and brain chemistry and causes several types of personality changes. As neurotransmitters decline, alcohol withdrawal and the symptoms associated with quitting after being a chronic alcohol drinkers are more painful becoming more prone to withdrawal symptoms that for the most part are symptoms of neurotransmitter malfunction or deficiency. The following chart is similar to the National Institutes For Health, chart that illustrates what neurotransmitters do but I've added the amino acids needed to produce the individual Neurotransmitters and neuropeptides peptides and to help lessen withdrawal type symptoms.

The following chart is an example, however, alcohol affects the brain in so many other ways, many ways are still unknown but these are a few examples regarding the basic neurotransmitters.

	NEUROTRANSMITTERS	
Neurotransmitter	Role In The Body	Alcohol Effect
Acetylcholine	Excitatory neurotransmitter used by the spinal cord neurons to control muscles and communicate through many neurons in the brain regulating memory.	Burns up acetylcholine fast triggering short burst feel good high then forms ill effects of acetaldehyde in the liver
Dopamine (Precursor amino-acid L-Tyrosine)	Inhibitory neurotransmitter produces feelings of pleasure when released by the brain reward systems. The body's natural cocaine.	Loss of dopamine causes hangover depression, Jittery motor function, mood, arousal
GABA (gamma-aminobutyric acid) (precursor amino-acid)	The major inhibitory neurotransmitter in the brain.	Loss of inhibitions
Glutamate (an amino-acid and neurotransmitter)	Excitatory brain neurotransmitter	Loss of motivation lethargic relaxant effect

Glycine (is an amino-acid neurotransmitter)	Inhibitory neurotransmitter used mainly by spinal cord, Motor function, eye function	Scattered thinking. Blurred or double vision, Loose slumped posture muscle relaxant
Norepinephrine (precursor amino-acid L-Tyrosine)	Excitatory Fight or Flight, action hormone regulator Arousal, attention, anxiety	Aggressive, combative, paranoia, fear.
Serotonin (precursor amino-acid L-Tryptophan)	Inhibitory pain, sensory perception, mood, appetite, alertness, sleep level of depression, aggression, and pain sensitivity	Hallucinations, Anger, Numbing effect of withdrawal and pain
Epinephrine (precursor amino-acid L-Tyrosine)	Adrenaline, is a hormone and neurotransmitter produced by the adrenal glands to increase heart rate, muscle strength, blood pressure and sugar metabolism.	Strong emotions such as fear or anger

Alcohol's Effect on Neurotransmitters

After drinking alcohol it crosses the blood-brain barrier. When alcohol is consumed it affects the production of many Neurotransmitters and block neuro pathways and the functioning of the bodily systems they regulate. The main neurotransmitters affected are:

- GABA,
- Glutamate,
- Serotonin,
- Dopamine,
- Endorphins.

Alcohol is an agonist for:

- GABA,
- Serotonin,
- Dopamine,
- Endorphins–it increases their activity.

Alcohol is an antagonist for glutamate, the main excitatory neurotransmitter, as it reduces glutamate activity and alcohol molecules affect the neurotransmitter system of dopamine.

Importance Of Neurotransmitter Support When You Quit

During Sobriety, a major step to successful recovery is assisting your brain and body in producing neurotransmitters again, naturally. It is an important part of preventing withdrawal symptoms such as headache, pain, confusion, muscle coordination and more withdrawal symptoms during rehab and preventing relapse in sobriety.

Low GABA- GABA deficiency in the brain and body can result in:

- Anxiety.
- Chronic stress.
- Depression.
- Difficulty concentrating and memory problems.
- Muscle pain and headaches.
- Insomnia and other sleep problems.

Low Serotonin Serotonin Deficiency may cause a range of psychological and physical symptoms. Serotonin deficiency is thought to be associated with several psychological symptoms, such as:

- Agitation
- Aggressive Behavior
- Anxiety or Feeling Anxious
- Depressed mood or sad
- Forgetfulness and Poor memory
- Impulsive behavior
- Irritability
- Irrational behaviors
- Poor appetite
- Self-esteem issues
- Sleep disturbance or Insomnia

Serotonin- The pineal gland produces serotonin. The precursor to melatonin is serotonin, a neurotransmitter that itself is derived from the amino acid tryptophan in the pineal gland serotonin is acetylated and then methylated to yield melatonin.

Low Serotonin- Physical symptoms Given its role in many of your body's vital functions, serotonin deficiency may also cause several physical symptoms, including:

- Carbohydrate/Sugar Cravings
- Increased Appetite/Weight Gain
- Fatigue/Poor Sleep
- Nausea
- Digestive Problems/IBS/Constipation

Dopamine- Dopamine is the main neuroendocrine inhibitor of the secretion of prolactin from the anterior pituitary gland. Dopamine produced by neurons in the arcuate nucleus of the hypothalamus is released in the hypothalamo hypophyseal blood vessels of the median eminence, which supply the pituitary gland.

Low Dopamine- The symptoms of a dopamine deficiency depends on the underlying cause. For example, a person with Parkinson's disease will experience very different symptoms from someone with low dopamine levels due to drug use. Some signs and symptoms of conditions related to a dopamine deficiency include:

- Jittery muscles, cramps, spasms, or tremors
- Body and headaches and pains
- Tight or stiff muscles
- Vertigo or loss of balance
- Bowel problems or constipation
- Cough or choking feeling, difficulty eating and swallowing
- Weight fluxuations lose or weight gain
- Heartburn or gastroesophageal reflux disease (GERD)
- Colds or frequent pneumonia
- Insomnia or trouble sleeping
- Fatigue or low energy
- Foggy mind or an inability to focus
- Slowed motor skills, moving or speaking more slowly than usual
- Tired or feeling of having no energy
- Unmotivated or feeling demotivated
- Mood feeling down, low sad and tearful
- High and low mood swings
- Despair or feeling hopeless
- Down on yourself or having low self-esteem
- Guilty feeling or guilt-ridden
- Anxiety or feeling anxious
- Thousgs of suicide or thoughts of self-harm
- No libido or lowered sex drive
- Hallucinating
- Delusional thinking
- Lack self-awareness

Low Endorphin Levels

Endorphins are naturally produced in response to pain. This phenomenon happens in both the Central Nervous System (CNS) and the Peripheral Nervous System (PNS). Endorphins are opiate like natural pain killers that are produced naturally in the body. When we get hurt or experience pain the body quickly releases these substances in the body so that we can better tolerate pain, childbirth and injury so they numb pain signals to a great extent. There are 4 types of endorphins are created in the human body. They are named:

1. Alpha Endorphins
2. Beta Endorphins
3. Gamma Endorphins
4. Sigma Endorphins

The 4 types of endorphins have different types of amino acids in their molecule. In the PNS, endorphins, primarily beta-endorphins, are released from the pituitary gland and bind to gamma-receptors. They are a pain relieving group of Neurotransmitters and neuropeptides that hinder neuro pathways produced by the endocrine system in the body. Endorphin deficiency isn't well understood. In general, if your body isn't producing enough endorphins, you might experience:

- depression
- anxiety
- moodiness
- aches and pains
- addiction
- trouble sleeping
- impulsive behavior

Alcohol Poisoning - Hangover & Ethanol Toxin Metabolism

Ethanol is the main alcohol found in beer, wine, and spirits and as ethanol is metabolised it creates a toxic compound known as acetaldehyde. A hangover is basically symptoms of acetaldehyde poisoning. Our bodies are 60% water so when we drink ethanol the molecules are quickly absorbed into our stomach and small intestines. Once the ethanol hits the bloodstream the ethanol moves throughout our entire body rapidly affecting the brain, nervous system, organ and musculoskeletal systems. The next phase of ethanol metabolism is an enzymatic oxidation process and there are two hepatic liver enzymes that are required to metabolise ethanol, ADH1B converts the ethanol to acetaldehyde and then ADH2 converts acetaldehyde to acetic acid. Acetaldehyde is one of the chemicals that is a major contributor responsible for symptoms of a hangover. Acetaldehyde is toxic to our body and it is therefore important that it gets further oxidized to acetic acid as quickly as possible. When there is not enough ADH2, and acetaldehyde builds up in the chemistry, it causes vasodilation and flushing of the skin and it is why we experience headaches and other unpleasant effects of a hangover. How bad the hangover is largely depends on how quickly our body biologically transmutates acetaldehyde to a vinegar like, acetic acid and eliminates it. Drinking too many alcoholic drinks too quickly results in more acetaldehyde in our body than can be broken down, thus causing alcohol poisoning and hangover syndrome. A hangover is an overload buildup of acetaldehyde due to inadequate enzymes that cannot metabolize the acetaldehyde into acetic acid quickly enough causing a chain reaction of symptoms associated with a hangover and alcohol poisoning. Alcohol poisoning can lead to death.

Blood Alcohol

A serving size of hard liquor is one jigger, or one ounce. A serving size of wine is five ounces. A beer is 10-12 ounces. The average person's BAC would be 0.02-.059 with one drink. The more servings you drink, the greater the impact the alcohol has on your body. Alcohol researchers have determined the BAC levels and alcohol poisoning symptoms as they start to show as follows:

- 0.02-0.039% – No loss of coordination, mild euphoria, minimization of shyness. Relaxation sets in.
- 0.04-0.059% – Feelings of well-being and relaxation, inhibitions lower, sensations of warmth. Euphoria takes hold. Minor impairment of judgment, memory, and lower caution.
- 0.06-0.99% – Slight impairment of balance, hearing, speech, vision, and reaction time. Lowered judgment and self-control. Impairment to reasoning and memory.
- 0.10-0.129% – Significant impairment of motor coordination and absence of good judgment. Slurred speech may start. Balance, peripheral vision, and hearing are impaired.
- 0.13-0.159% – Gross motor impairment. Lack of physical control. Vision is blurred and balance is difficult. Euphoria reduces and dysphoria (a feeling of being unwell) begins to set in.
- 0.160-0.199% – Dysphoria takes over and nausea sets in. This is the "sloppy drunk" point.
- 0.20-0.249% – Ability to walk is significantly diminished, absolute mental confusion. Nausea and vomiting. Possible blackout.
- 0.250-0.399% – Alcohol poisoning. Potential loss of consciousness.
- 0.40%+ – Onset of coma, possible death due to respiratory arrest.

Alcohol poisoning begins shutting down your organ systems at 0.20 It is possible to accidentally reach alcohol poisoning fast if you drink quickly when consuming a number of drinks more quickly than your body can metabolize them. Over 2,200 people die yearly from alcohol poisoning many of them are not alcoholics and some are new to drinking alcohol.

Appearance Of An Alcohol Drinker

Alcohol is a toxin and negatively affects your physical and mental appearance and most of the ways aren't pretty or attractive. The appearance of being inebriated or under the influence of alcohol might include:

- False Courage / Liquid Courage -
- Aggressive behavior and actions
- Blood shot eyes
- Slurred Speech
- Clumsy, staggering, or an unsteady gait
- Smell of alcohol on the breath
- Loss of bladder control pissing themself
- Mood-swings / behavior changes excessive laughter or crying
- Black out- unconscious behavior, anger, belligerent or loud talk
- Crazy Talk- Irrational thinking.
- Vomiting - violent body rejection of poison
- Crying and laughing (alternating)- pent up emotional releases
- Excessive use of mouthwash, breath mints, gum or cologne
- Avoidance of contact- avoiding people to hide a drinking problem
- Sedated or Sedentary - no energy, lethargic
- Sleeping at odd times - passing out
- Depressant- feeling sad from withdrawal of serotonin in the brain

The list of signs are signals that someone is using alcohol but does not mean that someone is an alcoholic. However, when there are performance and conduct problems coupled with any number of these signs an alcohol problem may be developing.

Anhedonia In Withdrawal

Some experts are of the opinion that Anhedonia does not exist however, several other research study authors suggest that anhedonia is a part of the abstinence withdrawal symptomatology and it is an important factor involved in relapse. When anhedonia is present in alcohol addicts somatoform disorders are possible and they can display symptoms that prevent the development of depressive state that interrupt normal healthy sexual desire and function, reduces enthusiasm for life, impaires ability to relate with other people, and weakens feelings of joy, affection, love, pride and self-respect. Protracted withdrawal is usually described as depression. However, Anhedonia displays additional mental and physical symptoms, such as feeling off, in a fog, with headache or fullness in the head, stomach pains, cravings, feelings of despair all are symptoms that may be caused by a functional deficit of dopamine transmission in the dopaminergic reward system after alcohol is abstained by an alcohol addicted individual and it can last up to a year. Physical anhedonia, is when you don't enjoy physical sensations, such as, receiving a hug that leaves you feeling empty rather than nurtured. Your favorite food taste bland and you may have a loss of appetite. It is important to do activities that give you a feeling of joy and happiness during rehab as it will help offset some of these negative withdrawal feelings. There are natural medicine, physio-therapeutic, psychotherapy and pharmacological treatment options available for the relief of the symptoms of Anhedonia however, various pleasant sensations can also, improve anhedonia and depression.

Alcohol and Sex

Alcohol is a tool of seduction, it reduces your inhibitions and makes you more open to engage in sexual behaviors that may not occur otherwise and may make a person unconscious and in a position where a predator could take advantage of you and coerce a person into unwanted sex. On the flip, alcohol also is linked to sexual dysfunctions and impotency, as well. While most decent people wouldn't have sex with a person that is unconscious, it's an open door of opportunity for a sexual predator who will pounce on the chance to take advantage of their victim. Alcohol is regularly used by sexual predators to spike an alcoholic beverage with a roofie, roponal or other date rape drugs. Alcohol can leave a person completely incapacitated and unable to consent to sex and it is the number one date-rape drug involved in 90% of all rapes. Even if you do consent to sex while under the influence of alcohol, you may not be safe about it. Therefore, you put yourself at risk for an unwanted and unplanned pregnancy and puts the baby at higher risk of birth defects. Alcohol increases risk for contracting a sexually transmitted (STD) disease. Intimacy is a sacred thing that is healthy when it is appropriately shared amongst consciously aware, loving and willing individuals and the pleasant feelings can release oxytocin during orgasm which is one of the pleasant sensations can help relieve and improve both c symptoms during alcohol recovery.

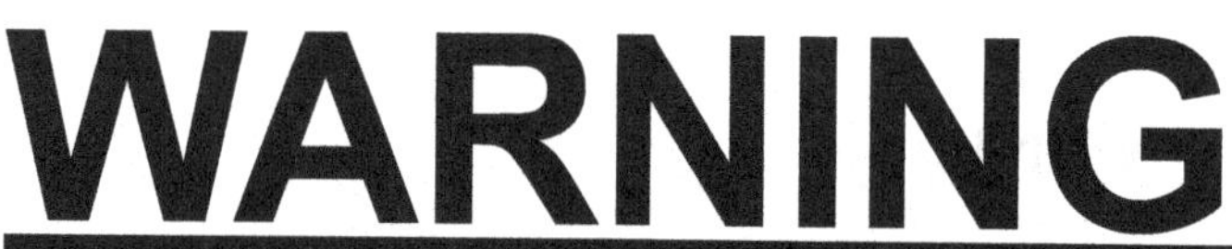

After The Consumption of
ALCOHOL
You May Wake Up Wondering What
The Heck Happened To You & Your Clothes!

Alcoholic Blackout

After a night of drinking you wake up and you have amnesia of the events prior to your awakening. This is called an "Alcoholic Blackout" episode. You are not alone many people who drink alcohol have probably done something they regretted while under the influence, at one point. During a blackout, basically, you remember drinking the night before but at some point, it all becomes a blur and you have no recollection of any of the events until the next day when you wake up. You may not even remember what happened, where you went or what you did. You may wake up in the presence of a stranger. In an unfamiliar place. In an unsafe environment. In a situation you don't want to be in, like jail. An alcoholic blackout leaves you without memory. Even if you do have a vague memory of what transpired, your left wondering what else happened that you don't remember. During a blackout, you wake up with regret. You do things during a blackout that is not acceptable behavior for anyone, like putting your cigarette out in your friends face instead of the ashtray. During a blackout, you may feel like you can drive but then you wake up in the hospital from crashing your car into a tree. What seemed like a good idea while you were drinking the night before may not seem so great in the morning light. After a blackout, you may have to do a lot of apologizing to the people you offend.

Alcohol Blackout Belligerent, Aggression & Violence

During an alcoholic blackout, people can become aggressive or belligerent and you may have to do a lot of apologising the next day after the booze wears off because you may not remember calling your jewish girlfriend a natzi bitch, when she tried to take away your keys. You may not remember calling your brother a bastard in front of your mother when you came home drunk. You could even wake up to find yourself jobless and you may not remember why? Pulling your pants down and telling your boss he's an asshole and that they can kiss your ass, usually, will get a person fired. You may even be embarrassed about your actions the night before, and you still have to repair relationships with people whom you upset while drinking. However, the damage can go beyond verbal assault, in fact, it gets much worse and Alcohol can make you do things and cause damage that no apology can repair. Most physical assaults, murders and homicides occur while people are under the influence of alcohol. Each year, there are more than three-million cases of violent crime traceable to alcohol use in America, specifically, homicide, sexual assault and domestic violence. Alcohol is involved in the majority of violent incidents. Among inmate populations, 80% have a history of abusing drugs or alcohol and about half are clinically addicted. Alcohol is a killer that ruins and ends lives.

Alcohol Lands People Behind Bars And In Graves

If you have had an alcoholic blackout and lived through it, consider yourself lucky, and take it as a final warning sign that is time to quit! Don't risk your future and the lives of others. If you have had an alcoholic blackout, your drinking has gone beyond being out of control. If it happens once, it will happen again and you may not be so lucky as to come out of it alive, next time and even if you do, you may end up losing someone you love or costing someone else their life and losing your freedom. Seek counseling and set boundaries for yourself and never put anyone in that situation again. Quit!

Alcohol and Drug Use

We live in a culture that encourages us to suppress our feelings and emotions. Alcohol consumption is driven by emotion. Alcohol stunts your emotional growth. Alcohol kills brain cells. We live in a society that it is unacceptable to express our anger. Some people think it is ok to express anger as long as we do not display negative emotions while doing so. There is a fine line between expressing these passionate emotions in a healthy manner as long as we do not cross the line of expressing anger abusively toward others. People are taught to swallow their tears and suppress their emotions, especially anger. We are all taught to wear a poker face and never raise our voice. The only place where it is acceptable to scream is at a ballgame and in fact, sports have been deliberately used to deflate man's aggression for a millennium as a method of keeping societies under control by the rulers. Boys are taught not to cry and told they are weak if they cry so men feel they are not even allowed to cry because it is perceived to be a sign of weakness. Give all the men sports and alcohol, that will keep them pacified and docile. That way of thinking is outdated and quite frankly, barbaric. It is ok for all of us to cry when the emotion hits us, let it out, have a good cry, express yourself with the most kindness possible to resolve and get back to your business. If you think about it no wonder 84.3 % of the population is on psychiatric drugs and 70% drink. This also means at least 15% of the population are dangerously drinking while taking psychiatric medications and many others are taking street drugs and alcohol which increases risk of fatalities. Mixing alcohol and drugs can kill you.

- Mixing antidepressants with alcohol increases depression and risk for developing an alcohol use disorder and can be deadly.
- Mixing cocaine with alcohol increases the risk of heart attack, violent outburst and sudden death.
- Consuming cocaine and alcohol together produces cocaethylene, a highly toxic substance that kills, over time as liver enzymes decline the greater the risk of death.
- Mixing antibiotics with alcohol reduces the effect of the antibiotic and an infection can kill. Additionally, some antibiotics can cause nerve damage when mixed with alcohol. Many antibiotics cause dizziness and drowsiness and alcohol makes the effects worse.
- Many over the counter medications can cause medical emergencies and even death if mixed with alcohol. Sleep aids, pain medications and cold remedies contain drugs that cannot safely be mixed while drinking alcohol.

Alcohol Use Is Self Harming Behavior

We have to take a different approach to how we view emotions in our society. To stay healthy we have to find a positive way to prevent stressful life situations by taking measures to heal our emotional health. There are many healthy ways to release those emotions instead of swallowing them down with pills and alcohol. Alcohol use itself is a self-harming behavior but unlike a cutter, cutting themself the physical damage is not visible, it is internal and behavioral. If we were taught to acknowledge and accept the importance of our emotional health there wouldn't be an alcohol epidemic or so many people lashing out in negative ways that create self-harm to themselves or harm to others. Our emotions must be expressed but not in a violent way such as shouting at someone or kicking the dog. Americans are in an emotional health crisis, and we have not found the solution, yet. You can't drink away your emotional wounds, but rather than suppressing them, it's better and healthier to go out in nature and shout at a tree and have a good cry and then hug the tree and apologize to the tree, than to try to drink emotional pain away.

Let it out but don't take it out on others

Alcohol Crutch For Emotional Pain or Illness

If we take a closer look at the alcohol abuser, we find that the feelings that drive alcoholism, we would find that many of us go to great measures to avoid those same emotions that trigger substance abuse. It is pain and the fear of pain, be it physical, emotional, mental or psychological that drives us to mind altering forms of substance abuse. Many drink away their tears instead of developing better interpersonal skills and since alcohol is numbing, it blocks people from expressing their emotions and feelings in a healthy manner causing an emotional constipation of sorts. The average human cries 10 gallons of tears in an average lifetime. Crying is a healthy means of releasing psychological grief. When you quit drinking, you will have a release of all the tears you've held back, it is better for your emotional health, to cry those tears than drink them away.

Many Drink Away Their Tears

People do not want to experience fear, they have anxiety and they drink it away. All the while, all those bottled up emotions are building up to an explosive level. Some alcohol drinkers drink as a subconscious way to be able to release their tears and emotions. People do not want to feel pain, be it emotional pain or physical pain drinkers can temporarily numb themself up with alcohol. Pain is part of the human condition be it child birth or injury. We want pain relief be it natural or chemically induced.

Alcohol Use Feelings of Despair People often drink alcohol to numb their feelings. Feelings of abandonment, loss, abuse, guilt, estrangement, rejection, low self-esteem, lack of self-worth, and shaming are the factors that cause self-destructive behaviors such as alcohol abuse. Many people who feel desperate or are feeling in despair, view alcohol as a quick emotional and physical pain reliever. Also, victims of verbal abuse will cope with living in an abusive relationship by drinking. Victims of bullying and shaming, will self-medicate emotional pay by drinking to forget their problems, swallow their pride, guilt and shame. Talking to a counselor is a healthier option who will help you find a real solution.

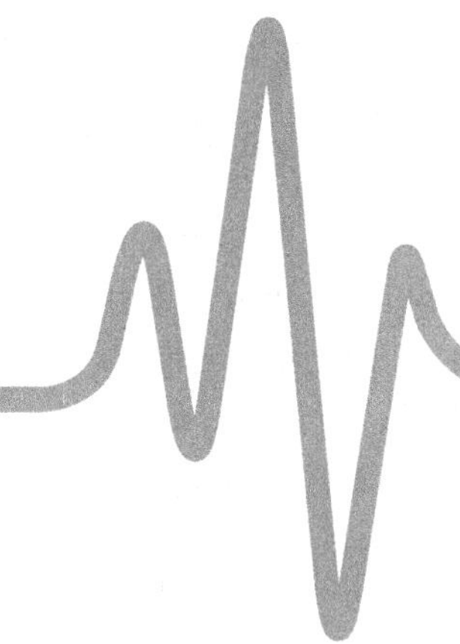

Chapter 4

Top Reasons People Drink

Why has alcohol abuse has become an epidemic in our lifetime? There are many factors that can contribute to alcoholism, and these are some reasons that are both environmental and genetic. People are more likely to become alcoholics when:

- They have repressed or unresolved emotional pain, fear or grief.
- They have a compulsive disorder and inclination to drink
- They associate drinking as a way to cope with pain or emotions
- They have been conditioned to drink alcohol during life's celebrations
- They reward themselves for a job well done with alcohol
- They view Alcohol as a treat, like a desert.
- They have a reason to drink on every occasion
- They don't have any reasons not to drink
- They have suppressed deep emotional wounds
- They have a close relative who is an alcoholic
- They were never taught healthy coping skills
- They learned poor coping or interpersonal skills
- They frequently face high-stress situations
- They struggle with anxiety and other emotions
- They live in a culture where alcohol is both used and accepted
- They lived in a home that alcohol use was permitted or encouraged
- They have a mental health condition, such as depression or bipolar
- Alcohol is readily available as a self-medicating vise

Alcohol 1st Anesthetic In History

People have searched for ways to alleviate and escape pain since the beginning of human existence. Alcohol is the oldest known sedative and it was used in ancient Mesopotamia thousands of years ago. In as early as 3400 BC, in the most ancient pharmacopeia in history, the Sumerians made wine as medicine and cultivated opium poppy as it is inscribed in the cuneiform tablets that were found in excavations of Nippur. In ancient India, in ayurvedic medicine it was common to use wine with incense of cannabis for anesthesia, after Arab traders brought it to India and China. However, the first I.V. anesthesia in modern medicine was an injection of opium with alcohol into a dog in Oxford in 1656, leading to the development of modern anesthesia. Also, from 1200-1500 AD, dwAle was an alcohol-based mixtured of bile, opium, lettuce bryony, henbane, hemlock and vinegar. In the U.S. during the civil war, a myth was that wounded soldiers would bite on a bullet during surgery but surgeons did in fact, anesthetize patients to render them unconscious during surgical procedures using Ether or Chloroform. Ether is made by distilling a mix of ethanol alcohol and sulphuric acid. Chloroform is an organic compound and is usually created by the chlorination of ester alcohol. The surgical gas anesthetic we use today is created by the chlorination of ester alcohol or methane. People anesthetize themselves with alcohol because they don't want to feel hurt and don't know how to deal with their pain. Alcohol was actually the very first anesthetic. Alcohol is the oldest known sedative; it was used in ancient Mesopotamia thousands of years ago.At some point, they took drank something and it made their painful problems temporarily go away. The euphoria and numbing effect that the alcohol gave them a false sense of relief. Alcohol numbs the body, the pain they had momentarily eliminated with alcohol returns and coming down from alcohol causes more intense pain than before they began using alcohol as an easy over-the-counter fix as a pain medication option that they can control. The truth is the alcohol is in control.

Alcohol #1 Use - Self-Medicating Pain

We are a culture in the middle of a pain epidemic. Ten percent of adults report having a drug or alcohol addiction at one point in their life; that's 23.5 million Americans. Studies show that just over two-thirds of our adult population (70.7 percent) are either overweight or obese. If many of these people are using food such as sugar as a drug. Sugar has a similar effect as alcohol in the body. Sugar can convert to alcohol in the body. Many cocktails are loaded with sugar and excess sugar turns into fat in the body. Alcohol adds many empty calories to your diet and it increases your appetite so you may end up gaining extra weight from drinking alcohol, too. Just as their are emotional eaters there are also emotional drinkers.

Many Eat & Drink Away Their Pain

Nearly three-quarters of the population are self-medicating by drinking or eating away their pain. There is a condition called, emotional eating disorder, and therefore there is also emotional drinking disorder. This is a staggering number, that continues to grow. We are all vulnerable to this type of self-medicating behavior, we are missing the root cause of alcohol abuse. Statistically, men drink more than women period. Men are antagonised to hold their emotions inside and the culture view men who cry as being weak. The reasons men drink more are related to the suppression of emotions and undiagnosed or mistreatment of mental health symptoms and conditions. It is important that we take a new less critical look at the state of mental health that cause so many of us to self-medicate with substances including alcohol.

Alcohol Liquid Courage

America prides itself on bravery, yet, Americans drink away their worries more than any other culture and alcohol abuse is rampant. Alcohol isn't instant courage it is more like temporary insanity. It takes courage to abstain from alcohol and those who do are the real courageous ones. America is the land of the free and home of the brave.

Many Drink Away Their Fears...

Self-medicating with alcohol is a poor mental health approach. Massive failure of medical misdiagnosis of alcohol use disorders, is partially the problem.

Psychological Pain, Mental Disorders and Alcohol Use

Psychological wounds can't be seen as well as physical wounds but they can be equally or sometimes even more damaging in a person's life. Psychological wounds are the hardest to heal and they are what drives people to drink, the most. Additionally, people with brain chemistry imbalances are more negatively affected by alcohol than those with normal brain chemistry. Alcohol is a no-no as is the case with most mental illness medications. Around 450 million people currently suffer from mental health conditions. The 5 most common mental health disorders include depression, anxiety, eating disorders, substance abuse and attention deficit disorder ADD/ADHD. Therefore, mental disorders are among the lead cause of ill-health disabilities, globally. There are various treatments available, however, only 2/3 of mentally ill people ever seek help from a health professional and many self-medicate with alcohol or other drugs. For example, about 1 in 100 people have schizophrenia and can have a variety of symptoms, such as hallucinations, delusions, hearing voices in their head or disordered behaviors. Additionally, they may have "negative" symptoms such as talking to themselves and imaginary others, delusional thoughts and problems in expressing their emotions. The cause of schizophrenia is not known but is usually onset in young adulthood between ages 16 and 30 and may have contributing factors, such as genetic, environment, and an altered brain chemistry and brain structure may play a role. Like most other mental health disorders the conventional treatment for schizophrenia is usually long-term psychiatric medications, such as, antipsychotic medication. Counseling is the most important treatment for mental illness and a nutritional approach is important regardless of conventional treatment and may help improve both positive and negative symptoms and also can help reduce the negative side-effects of medication.

The following nutrition tips that may be helpful:

- Cease consuming alcohol.
- Correct blood sugar problems
- Eat a healthy diet

- Avoid excess stimulants, caffeine or drug use
- Supplement essential fatty acid imbalances - Omega 3, 6 & 9
- Increasing antioxidants; niacin (Vitamin B3) therapy
- Addressing methylation problems helped by B12 and folic acid
- Lab test brain chemistry, pyroluria and supplement zinc
- Identify and eliminate food allergies

Anxiety is the number one mental disorder and many try to calm their anxious nerves and nervous energy with alcohol but because it is a depressant it may cause dangerous mood swings. People who are depressed become more depressed and some even become suicidal under the influence of alcohol. People with emotional issues and wounds are also at a higher risk of the negative effects of alcohol. People with anger issues, jealousy and betrayal issues are at higher risk to commit violent crimes while under the influence of alcohol and are more likely to have violent episode which result in assaults and homicide. Alcohol in general, lowers inhibitions in people, and the worst behaviors and personalities are more likely to come out while under the influence of alcohol and other drugs. Most people can get crazy-drunk and do stupid things while under the influence of alcohol. All people get a depressive hangover even after mild drinking because alcohol is a depressant.

Alcohol Mask Mental Illness

The system has been set to just throw the alcoholic addict into a dry tank and let the criminal justice system deal with the drunks. This may be an obstacle that prevents mental health care system from delivering the proper care for those suffering from alcohol use disorder. There is a shortage of mental healthcare treatment facilities for dual diagnosis alcohol use disorders. Many who are thrown in jail for DUI's should be admitted into a substance abuse mental health program, instead. Additionally, there is a lack of public health awareness campaigns and government ran treatment centers have a growing necessity for the masses to effectively resolve the alcohol disease epidemic. The lack of effective public health anti-alcohol awareness campaigns is a contributing factor that is killing so many, due to alcohol abuse.

Solution To The American Alcohol Binge

There is an Alcohol use epidemic. 32 million Americans struggle with a drinking problem. Alcohol is the #1 breakup & divorce drug used but you can't drink away your heartache or drown your sorrows with alcohol for very long because it is an emotion numbing depressant that only makes you feel even more emotionally empty. Alcohol is a poor choice as a coping tool, filling your belly and numbing your feelings with Alcohol never solved anyone's problems, it only prolongs them and makes them worse. Many people think they are going out to drink a few drinks and have a good time, but end up in an Alcohol induced hell filled with legal problems, DUI's, fines, jail time, job or relationship loss and more disasters. Alcohol destroys lives and futures. Don't let Alcohol turn your dream life into a nightmare. Quit or Die offers a solutions to help you:

- Break Up With Alcohol and Feel More Love In Relationships
- Live A Longer and Happier Life
- Find Lost Motivation & Feel More Energy

Why Are Wine, Beer & Cocktails Bad? What level of regular drinking is safe? Why read Quit or Die? It brings awareness about the following:

- Alcohol Accelerates Aging
- Alcohol Antioxidants Are Not An Anti-Aging Potion
- Alcohol is Dehydrating and Dries Your Skin Out Like A Prune
- Alcohol Shortens Your Lifespan
- That Extra Glass of Wine Cost You 1/2 Hour Off Your Life
- Chugging A Picture Of Beer = 2 Years Off Your Life
- Alcohol Makes You Look Older Quicker

There is nothing healthy, sexy, romantic or glamorous about drinking. Alcohol Ad Campaigns show happy attractive people drinking and having a good time but these ads are deceptive and are skillfully designed to brain-wash you and tempt you into drinking. The truth is, Alcohol robs you of your health, motivation and energy while it slowly sucks the life out of you! Alcohol is toxic. 13.8 million Americans are alcoholics. Alcohol is a body-snatcher, that claimed the lives of 88,000 fellow Americans, last year.

Quit or Die helps you:

- Curb Alcohol Cravings Safely & Effectively
- Kick Your Alcohol Affair To The Curb
- Be Closer To Your Loved Ones
- Get Your Energy and Motivation Back
- Slow Aging & Feel Younger

Bringing Alcohol Problems To Work

According to the National Institute on Alcohol Abuse and Alcoholism (NIAAA), nearly 14 million Americans abuse alcohol, that is 1 in every 13 adults, abuse alcohol or are alcoholics. Several million more adults engage in risky drinking behaviors that can progressively, lead to alcohol dependency problems. The costs of alcohol damages to society in terms of lost productivity, loss time off work, sick days that are taken for hangovers, loss of jobs, loss of income, loss of family relationships, loss of livelihood, health care costs, traffic accidents, and more personal tragedies are staggering.

Alcohol stays in your system for over 24 hours. Many may think they are sober in the morning after a night of a few drinks. In some cases the alcohol level is detectable at the start of the work day. In the workplace, the costs of alcoholism and alcohol abuse manifest themselves in many different ways. Absenteeism is estimated to be 4 to 8 times greater among alcoholics and alcohol abusers. Other family members of alcoholics also have greater rates of absenteeism from dealing with alcohol related crisis of their loved ones. If Alcohol use gets out of hand, it becomes a threat to everything in your life; your job, relationships, health, livelyhood and ultimately, your life.. Numerous studies and reports have been issued on the workplace costs of alcoholism and alcohol abuse, and they report costs that range from $33 billion to $68 billion per year. Alcohol increases risk of accidents in all environments work, home and in automobiles. Don't wait until you cause an accident to change, get help.

Employer Intervention Safety & Help Programs

Many companies offer an Employee Assistance Program. EAP's, offer its employees education and support to help deal with all kinds of problems in the workplace. If your company doesn't offer an EAP, call your local union and ask about EAP options. An EAP can be a first line of defense in getting help as EAP's provide short-term counseling, assessment, and referral of employees with alcohol and drug abuse problems, emotional and mental health problems, marital and family problems, financial problems, dependent care concerns, and other personal problems that can affect the employee's work performance in an attempt to help employees improve problems before they progress to a state of irreparable damages. These types of EAP services are confidential. The programs are usually staffed by professional counselors and may be operated in-house with agency personnel, under a contract with other agencies or EAP providers or a combination of the two. Accidents and on-the-job injuries are far more prevalent among alcoholics and alcohol abusers. Take advantage of these programs if you have them available on your job or find a good local support group outside before it cost your job.

Effects On The Job

Alcohol is the single most used and abused drug in America. According to the National Institute on Alcohol Abuse and Alcoholism (NIAAA), nearly 14 million Americans (1 in every 13 adults) abuse alcohol or are alcoholics. Several million more adults engage in risky drinking patterns that could lead to alcohol problems. The costs of alcohol to society in terms of lost productivity, health care costs, traffic accidents, and personal tragedies are staggering. Numerous studies and reports have been issued on the workplace costs of alcoholism and alcohol abuse, and they report costs that range from $33 billion to $68 billion per year.

Alcohol And Unemployment

Alcohol is a major factor in injuries, at home, at work and on the highway. In the workplace, the costs of alcoholism and alcohol abuse manifest themselves in many different ways. Absenteeism is estimated to be 4 to 8 times greater among alcoholics and alcohol abusers. Other family members of alcoholics also have greater rates of absenteeism. Accidents and on-the-job injuries are far more prevalent among alcoholics and alcohol abusers. Additionally, alcohol affects workers in other ways, too. According to the federal government's 2013 National Survey on Drug Use and Health, about 1 in 6 unemployed workers were addicted to alcohol or drugs which was twice the rate of full-time workers that were addicted, in that year. The latest survey showed that 17% of unemployed workers had a substance abuse disorder last year, whereas 9% of full-time workers did. If your company has an alcohol prevention program, get involved. The program can help you have success on your path to sobriety. For example, Operation RedBlock is a union-initiated, management-supported program that uses peer involvement to prevent employee use of alcohol and/or drugs while on the job. The program emphasizes safety awareness, education, and prevention of on the job alcohol and drug use. It is a peer accountability approach primarily employee-run substance abuse prevention and intervention plan that proven beneficial for many companies. Many companies offer similar programs that can be beneficial to your sobriety success. Get involved and help others, too.

Your Body and Alcohol

When a person is intoxicated, alcohol interferes with the ability to analyze sensory information and interferes with a person's ability to make sound rational decisions resulting in the symptoms of being drunk and other side effects including:

- Decrease and Loss motor coordination
- Off Balance or Dizzy
- Slurred Speech
- Blurred Vision
- Illogical thinking
- Sweating
- Mood Swings- from happy to Irritated and argumentative
- Loss of judgment- Loss of the ability to judge distance and heights
- Dulled sensation of pain
- Vomiting/Sick- bad reactions-
- Medication Interactions-alcohol does not mix well with medications.

Long-Term Health Damages

The liver breaks down the majority of the alcohol we drink, creating acetaldehyde as a byproduct. acetaldehyde, which is a carcinogenic, causes the liver to accumulate fat, according to Doug Simonetto, a hepatologist at the Mayo Clinic. Therefore, when you quit drinking you should also lose some weight from around your waist, automatically.

- Potentially fatal: high blood pressure, heart disease, stroke
- Cancers: breast, mouth, throat, esophagus, liver and colon
- Alcoholic hepatitis, liver disease and digestive problems
- Weight Gain & Obesity Related Conditions.

Alcohol Toxicity

Alcohol is a carcinogen. Alcohol is one of the most toxic substances to humans in existence. It's literally poisoning us when we feel drunk.A new study released in the journal Alcoholism suggests that cutting alcoholic drinks with diet soda makes them more potent than using their full-calorie counterparts. Specifically, researchers found that mixing alcohol with diet (sugar-free) soft drinks resulted in a higher breath alcohol content than mixing alcohol with a regular (sugar-sweetened) soft drinks. Diet sodas make the alcohol even more toxic because diet sodas are filled with chemicals and artificial sweeteners that also pose negative side effects and health risks. Mixing alcohol with diet soda compounds the toxicity level of the drink. Drink too much at once and you'll never wake up again. Drink too much over time and you could find yourself facing a host of medical problems, including cancer.

Todays alcohol is not what it used to be. Many of the grains are genetically modified. Corn for example, may have GMO, genetically modified organisms. Some GMO grains are modified to contain silkworm DNA to prevent live silkworms from damaging the crop. The silkworm is not a carnivore and wont eat its own DNA. However, not many people would willing drink alcohol if they knew what was in their drink, or that contains cross DNA of genetically modified organisms. Many grains used in making alcohol spirits are genetically modified and in some studies the human consumption of GMO's cause all kinds of disease and DNA damage in humans, including cancer.

Beer Is The Most Consumed Alcohol

Beer is the number one consumed alcoholic beverage and very few brands are non-GMO, most brands are loaded with various GMO grains which we have no idea of how they will interact inside the body during the digestive process. Beers top the charts at almost 200 calories a bottle, their are potentially trace amounts of herbicides and pesticides if the grains are not organically grown, not to mention all of the empty carbohydrates from the hops and barley. Herbicides and pesticides are endocrine disruptors that wreak havoc on your hormonal system. Even if you choose non-GMO brands, the other ingredients mixed into a typical cocktail is riddled with toxins, artificial colorings, artificial flavorings, and high fructose corn syrup. It takes your liver 51 days to digest a molecule of hydrogenated fat. High fructose, is poison also. It spikes the blood sugar and can cause blood sugar issues. Even if a cocktail was made "with all non-GMO ingredients and ingredients were labeled with full transparency your drink menu ingredient list would look something like this:

- 1.5 oz. Jigger of Tequila (Class 1 IARC Carcinogen)
- 2 oz. Margarita Mixer (glycol + artificial preservative- carcinogen)
- 1/4 cup Corn Simple syrup (high fructose corn syrup)
- 0.5 oz. Fresh Lemon Juice (Beta-limonene)
- 0.25 oz. Agave Nectar (Saponins)
- 2 Cilantro Leaves (Alpha-terpineol) trace pesticides
- 1 dash Jalapeno slices (Capsaicin)
- 1 cup club soda (phosphoric acid) (Aliphatic hydrocarbons)

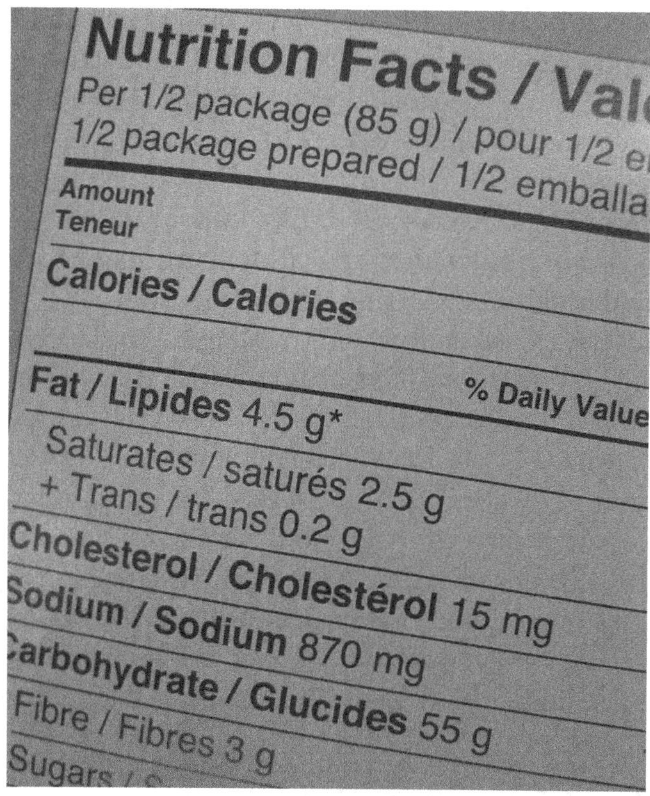

What Is In The Mix!

Even if it is low calorie, sugar free and GMO free drink mixer, those are not the most harmful things in some of the drink mixers. Mixed drinks contain many artificial ingredients, such as propylene glycol (PG) which is a byproduct of fossil fuel that is actually propane-1,2-diol a petro byproduct. Many additives and colorings are deemed safe in small amounts but potentially poisonous in larger quantities and may pose a risk when mixing multiple processed food and drink items and by consuming them together in a short period of time. In the process of making plastics from petroliates many compounds are formed one of them being propylene oxide which is considered a human carcinogen and it is the precursor to propylene glycol, yet PG is thought to be safe at the current time. The most alarming thing about PG, is that it accumulates in the human body over time, besides that, no one wants to hear something that is found in anti-freeze is in their drink mix. Keep in mind, this is only one example of many chemicals found in drink mixers. I first learned about propylene glycol when I was formulating the anti-aging brand skincare line, I decided not to include it as an ingredient as it increases your skin's propensity to absorb whatever it comes into contact with. Considering the large amount of other dangerous chemicals we encounter on a regular basis, that may be of even more danger than the PG compound itself. During my research of PG, I was super shocked to find out that it is used in some processed foods and drinks, as it helps keep liquids from separating. In my opinion, water is the most detoxifying and neutralizing compound on the planet and in the human body, so we don't want to be consuming a compound that may bind together toxins or hinder the body from separating and eliminating toxins from the body. According to the University of Connecticut study, propylene glycol toxicity can be dangerous for those with liver problems. Most every chronic drinker would want to protect their liver from this as it would pose a compounded risk to a drinker's liver. The CDC's toxicity profile of propylene glycol, negatively assessed it in neurological symptoms. When taken orally and tested by patch test, the amount of the chemical was found in the system of a number of test subjects who were found to have varying degrees of neurological issues, also, including stupor, convulsions and other unspecified severe mental symptoms. Regardless, if it is deemed safe, by the FDA, what is often overlooked is that it is hidden in many other processed foods and drinks and it is accumulative in the human body, overtime. Therefore, this is another reason to read product labels, avoid PG and quit drinking mixed alcoholic drinks made with mixers, sodas and flavored iced coffee if they contain PG. FDA has recently cracked down on the E-cigarette industry, which may bring more attention to the study of PG in humans, as one main ingredients used in electronic cigarettes is propylene glycol, PG is a synthetic liquid artificial smoke and it is also used to produce fog for fire-fighting trainings and to make fog on concert stages and theatrical productions. Lastly, in a cat-based study of the toxic effects of propylene glycol, cats receiving the high dose developed decreased activity, mental depression, and slight to moderate ataxia.

Alcohol Causes Cancer

Alcohol is a carcinogen. Drinking even one alcoholic drink per day is linked with a 5 % increase in the risk of breast cancer a 17 % increase in the risk of oropharyngeal throat cancer and a 30 % increase in the risk of esophageal cancer in comparison with not drinking.

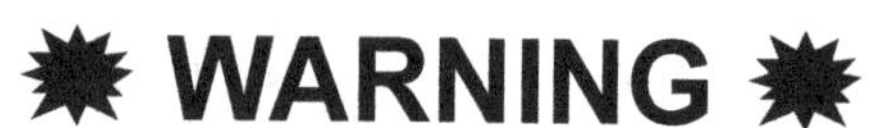

Drinking Distilled Spirits And Alcoholic Beverages Increase Your Risk Of Cancer And Alcohol May Cause Birth Defects During Pregnancy

Every bottle of alcohol is required to have a warning label informing the public of the proven health risks and consequences of drinking alcohol. Yet, many still drink it knowing it is a poison carcinogen that can destroy health and our lives. Additionally, alcohol does not mix well with chemotherapy and radiation treatments of cancer patients.

Alcohol Skin Aging

The negative effects of alcohol on your skin includes: dehydration, premature wrinkles, collagen decrease, volume loss, sagging skin from loss of elasticity, redness and blotchy skin. The amount and frequency of drinking determines the magnitude of the damage. Alcoholic drinks may cause early aging. Additionally, if you have a cut, scratch or other wound, do not pour rubbing alcohol on your skin, either, it prevents it from healing and it can make scars form or worsen as alcohol interrupts the healing processes.

Abuse Vs Dependance

Alcohol dependence, is an progressive disease state that causes:

- Craving - a strong need to drink alcohol
- Loss of control - not being able to stop drinking once you've started
- Physical dependence - withdrawal symptoms
- Tolerance - the need to drink more alcohol to feel the same effect

With alcohol abuse, you are not physically dependent, but you still have a serious problem. The drinking may cause problems at home, work, or school. It may cause you to put yourself in dangerous situations, or lead to legal, financial, relationship or social problems.

Long Term Health Effects of Alcohol

Alcoholism shortens a person's life expectancy by ten years, according to the New England Journal of Medicine. Alcohol causes accelerated aging, appetite loss, nerve disorders, nerve damage, brain damage, osteoporosis, depression, and muscle cramps.

Also, binge drinking leads to severe brain damage, blood clots and strokes. Health decline is an inevitable situation when a person drinks excessive alcohol. Additionally, alcohol is a diuretic that makes you urinate speeding up the loss of fluid from the body and causes dehydration if you fail to drink enough water. These are some other negative effects on your health.

- Dehydration is the reason that symptoms of a hangover, including headache, dizziness, thirst, paleness, and tremors are all caused by dehydrating effect of drinking too much alcohol. Long term alcohol consumption contributes to signs of aging, dry wrinkled skin, dry frizzy hair by chronic dehydration.
- Alcohol interrupts deep delta slow wave sleep levels, which is the state of sleep that repairs the body.
- Even though an over drinker may pass out or fall asleep it may appear as if they're in a deep sleep, but they are not getting restorative sleep.
- Consuming 5 or more alcoholic beverages in 1 night can affect your brain and body activities for up to 3 days.
- 2 consecutive nights of drinking 5 or more alcoholic beverages can affect your brain and body activities for up to 5 days.
- Your attention span is shorter for up to 48 hours after drinking.
- Depending on a person's individual metabolism, even the effects of small amounts of alcohol under the legal limit (BAC of .03) can still persist for a longer period of time than standard estimates.
- Permanent damage to the brain and bodily systems even after the acute effects of alcohol impairment disappear.

The "direct toxicity" of alcohol damages the nervous system from the brain down to the spinal cord and peripheral nerves.

Difference Between Alcoholism and Alcohol Abuse

There are tell tale signs that determine if someone is abusing alcohol or someone is suffering with alcoholism. Commonly the two conditions are confusing to tell apart. They are different and not the same. The main difference is seen in the symptoms of each one. Someone who suffers from alcoholism:

- Feels they need alcohol daily to function.
- Suffers withdrawal once alcohol level gets low in the body
- Progressively increases alcohol intake as tolerance levels rise.
- Can not drink in moderation or control the amount of alcohol
- Can not stop drinking.
- They will continue to drink no matter how hard they try not to.

An Alcohol Abuser:

- Has developed a small alcohol tolerance
- Suffers from minimal alcohol withdrawal when they are sober
- Neglects obligations to enable themselves to drink more often
- Will drink and drive
- Will drink alcohol to cope with emotional reactions
- Feels they have to drink to have a good time
- Will drink alcohol in excess
- Does not drink every day or feel the need to

The differences are subtle, but they are different. The greatest concern is denial. People who tend to believe that it will never happen to them and that they are safe from alcoholism. Denial makes one feel immune from alcoholism. Many do not worry much about their drinking and frequently abusing alcohol but it alcoholism can happen suddenly.

Research has shown that continued alcohol abuse will eventually result in alcoholism if the abuse is not stopped. Anyone who abuses alcohol long-term is at high-risk for becoming an alcoholic, even if they think they're in control.

Stages of Alcoholism

- **Early** - Regular Social or Occasional Drinking. Less than 2 alcohol use disorder symptoms.
- **Chronic** - ongoing nearly daily alcohol consumption with dependance the negative outcomes associated with alcohol use that has potentially devastating effects on one's life, including poor health, conflict in relationships, troubled finances. When abstaining, the drinker may experience anxiety, confusion, tremors, racing heart, nausea, vomiting, and/or sleeplessness.
- **Alcohol Abuse** - As the chronic alcohol use continues, alcohol abuse advances and six or more of the alcohol use disorder symptoms appear, this is the point indicating need for treatment intervention for addiction.
- **High Functioning Alcoholic** -however 20% of alcohol abusers are considered "highly functioning" and are able to work daily and meet their financial obligations but eventually negative alcohol related consequences appear in some way as their alcoholism advances.
- **End Stage Alcoholism** - In the end stage of alcoholism, instead of living to drink, the drinker, drinks to live. At this point, the drinker has lost control of their ability to stop drinking and they are usually suffering with physical illness and sick from their drinking.

After a long enough period, a heavy chronic alcohol users withdrawal symptoms may be so painful that the alcoholic is motivated to continually drink to prevent the painful symptoms of delirium tremens and sudden death by abstinence withdrawal. Worse yet, the drinker may love drinking and have no desire to quit, no matter what the consequence. This is mental illness and needs professional and usually institutionalised care.

Having The "Alcohol Problem" Talk

Approaching someone about their drinking problem requires a tactful approach. To tell someone they are an alcoholic is cruel, for it shames them profoundly. It is shameful to have to acknowledge that you are controlled by alcohol. Alcoholics are enbondaged to a drug, they are not free, they are a slave to a substance, they no longer have any control over, they have been defeated by the bottle and lower emotional impulses. To not say anything, to not try to help or to just leave someone in a state of drinking themselves to death, is much more cruel, and, in the end, will greatly increase the sum of suffering and misery for everyone in the life of the alcoholic. When a loved one drinks too much, at some point it has to be confronted, and the sooner the better. Denial is common and to come to a solution "having the talk" or an intervention to acknowledgement the truth is one of the first steps to recovery.

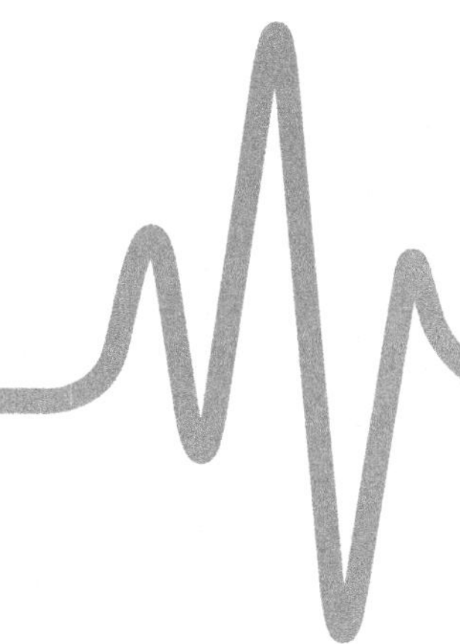

Chapter 5

BAC Limits by State

First of all, no one should ever even think of driving after drinking any amount. Even a minimum amount of Alcohol can stay in your system for up to 24 hours. Your blood alcohol level is what authorities will check with the BAC breathalyzer test during a field sobriety test to see if you measure over the states legal limit for drinking and driving. Many states have mandatory jail time for first time offenders. Wisconsin is the most lenient state and a first-offense isn't even a crime. It's a civil infraction that results in a ticket. This is likely why four cities in the state are amongst the highest in alcohol consumption in the nation. The following list the legal limits and the maximum BAC scores where they throw the book at DUI offenders with maximum punishment and zero tolerance of drinking and driving:

State	"Per Se" BAC Level	"Zero Tolerance" BAC Level	Enhanced Penalty BAC Level	
Alabama	.08	.02	—	
Alaska	.08	.00	.15	
Arizona	.08	.00	.15	
Arkansas	.08	.02	.15	
California	.08	.02	.16	

Colorado	.08	.02	.17	
Connecticut	.08	.02	.16	
Delaware	.08	.02	.15	
District of Columbia	.08	.00	.15	
Florida	.08	.02	.15	
Georgia	.08	.02	.15	
Hawaii	.08	.02	.15	
Idaho	.08	.02	.20	
Illinois	.08	.00	.16	
Indiana	.08	.02	.15	
Iowa	.08	.02	.15	
Kansas	.08	.02	.15	
Kentucky	.08	.02	.18	

Louisiana	.08	.02	.15	
Maine	.08	.00	.15	
Maryland	.08	.02	—	
Massachusetts	.08	.02	.20	
Michigan	.08	.02	.17	
Minnesota	.08	.00	.16	
Mississippi	.08	.02	—	
Missouri	.08	.02	.15	
Montana	.08	.02	—	
Nebraska	.08	.02	.15	
Nevada	.08	.02	.18	
New Hampshire	.08	.02	.18	
New Jersey	.08	.01	.10	

New Mexico	.08	.02	.16	
New York	.08	.02	.18	
North Carolina	.08	.00	.15	
North Dakota	.08	.02	.18	
Ohio	.08	.02	.17	
Oklahoma	.08	.02	.17	
Oregon	.08	.00	—	
Pennsylvania	.08	.02	.16	
Rhode Island	.08	.02	.15	
South Carolina	.08	.02	.16	
South Dakota	.08	.02	.17	
Tennessee	.08	.02	.20	
Texas	.08	.02	.15	

Utah	.05	.02	.16	
Vermont	.08	.02	—	
Virginia	.08	.02	.15	
Washington	.08	.02	.15	
West Virginia	.08	.02	.15	
Wisconsin	.08	.02	.15	
Wyoming	.08	.02	.15	

Laws vary from state to state, including the license suspension procedure and penalties upon conviction. No one should ever drink and drive. In 2016, 10,497 people died in alcohol-impaired driving crashes, accounting for 28% of all traffic-related deaths in the United States. Of the 1,233 traffic deaths among children ages 0 to 14 years in 2016, 214 (17%) involved an alcohol-impaired driver.

No Level of Drinking and Driving is Safe

Alcohol Field Sobriety Test (FST)

If you are pulled over an officer will likely conduct a field sobriety test (FST). This is typically why and how this test is conducted. There are 5 tests chosen to constitute the "Standardized Field Sobriety Tests", which are:

(1) the Horizontal Gaze Nystagmus Test;
(2 the Walk & Turn Test; walk a straight line.
(3 the One-Leg Stand Test
(4 touch the tip of the nose, arms outstretched finger tip to nose
(5 breathalyzer - blow to determine (BAC)

Although most law enforcement agencies continue to use a variety of these FSTs, most use the three-test battery of validated field sobriety tests, referred to as the Standardized Field Sobriety Test (SFST). The NHTSA-approved battery of tests consists of the Horizontal Gaze Nystagmus Test (HGN Test), the Walk-and-Turn Test (WAT), and the One-Leg-Stand Test (OLS). BAC is most accurate.

Alcohol Impairment

The mental and physical impairments as a result of drinking alcohol increases accident rates among alcohol drinkers is a direct result of the alcohol`s effects on the drinker's brain, thus, impairing the reflex responses, blurring vision and weakening muscle coordination further slowing down responses and reaction time in addition to negatively affecting judgment and therefore increases accident and injury risk to self and others. This is why you should never operate heavy equipment, mechanical machinery or drive while under the influence of alcohol. Even without alcohol, anyone can get in an accident, because to err is human. However, getting into an accident while under the influence of alcohol, will be deemed the drinkers fault even if the other person involved make the mistake or cause an accident, thus resulting in legal issues for the drinker.

Lawyers Alcohol Use

One of the first people a DUI offender will call is their lawyer. Lawyers are under constant pressure and are expected to solve everyone's problems. Lawyers are not immune to the Alcohol epidemic, either. The alcoholism rate for lawyers is 1- in-3 practicing lawyers is a problem drinker. Lawyers in practice for 10 years and less have significantly higher alcoholism rates than senior lawyers and 29% have a drinking problem. After that, for lawyers working in their second decade, the rate is 21 %. It is part of the legal professions culture, to drink. There is some belief that drinking problems start in law school, but at the same time, 44 % of lawyers in the study said their problematic drinking habits started in their initial 15 years of being in practice. There is a high rate of mental stress, mental problems and suicide in lawyers. Lawyers are 3.6 times more likely to suffer from depression. Clinical depression and substance abuse are highly correlated with suicide rates. The legal industry has the 11th-highest incidence of suicide. Many self-medicate with alcohol. This indicates that starting a legal career can be correlated with a high likelihood of developing a drinking problem.

Punishing Alcoholics As Criminals

Over 1.4 million drivers were arrested for DUIs in 2009 and rightfully so, no one should ever drink and drive. However, alcoholism is not an issue of stupidity and bad behavior, it is a disease. Everyone knows drunk driving is a crime, yet people do it. DUI's are expensive it cost up to $1,000.00. Going to jail for DUI is extremely life disrupting. If a person gets one DUI and does not learn the lesson not to drink and drive that person has serious problems. Drinking and driving and getting a 2nd DUI goes beyond making a stupid mistake and that person receives jail time up to a year behind bars plus the maximum fine is up to $10,000.00. Those who get ticketed for their 2nd DUI have more than a serious problem, statistically, this type of person has serious behavioral issues and likely more than one addiction problem. In addition, most have a psychological disorder, as well. This type of individual puts everything in their life and others at risk. Therefore, this type of alcohol abuser needs to undergo serious counseling and go into an institutionalised rehab. A repeat offender has established a proven track record of having a disregard for risking human lives and this legally becomes a criminal alcohol abuse problem that is beyond self-control. Repeat offenders are obviously, incapable of making rational decisions regarding controlling their behavior while under the influence of alcohol and need a psychological evaluation and treatment.

Over Half of American Inmates Are Incarcerated Due To Alcohol Related Crimes

Jail Health Care AWS

The Bureau of Justice Statistics estimates that 17,358 individuals in custody died during the period from 2007-2010. Studies show, many jails are not equipped to handle the medical emergencies of alcohol withdrawal syndrome such as DT's in jail. Many jail facilities do not have a treatment system set up to treat inmates with alcohol withdrawal syndrome AWS. The majority of inmates, who are alcoholics are at high risk of serious health complications and even death from DTs Delirium Tremens while in jail. It is not fair for the officers to be forced to deal with the special health care needs of alcoholics. Additionally, it is not fair to the alcoholic when often their civil rights are violated and they receive substandard care for alcohol withdrawal syndrome, while in custody from alcohol related crimes. We need another emergency system in place to handle those patients with blood alcohol levels bordering alcohol poisoning. A dry cell is a dangerous place for an alcoholic in DT's.

Inmates With Addiction

Alcohol is a legal drug and is easily accessible. Studies show, another set of alcohol abusers will continue risky drinking behaviors even after they get out of jail on a citation for public intoxication or DUI. Addiction is never about the alcohol. If it was, jails would work. The approach to take the drugs and alcohol out of the offenders environment and them returning to a functional state of mind, is only temporary, unless the offender is educated and motivated to quit. The system does little to truly recover the addict, and usually the addict will not stick to sobriety after release. If the addict had a sobriety lifestyle and a personal commitment to sobriety, then their lives would have a better chance at becoming manageable again. However, in reality, this rarely ever happens. It is not about the crime it is about addiction. If they are addicted, regardless of the criminal consequences they will stay addicted in the state of mind and to the physical effects.

Alcohol Increases Crime

Alcohol-related crime statistics reveal a close, intimate connection between alcohol and violence. On average, in any given year:

- 86 percent of homicides will be committed by individuals under the influence.
- 40 percent of child abuse incidents will be connected to alcohol use or abuse, and 70 percent of these abusive individuals (parents or guardians) will suffer from a substance use disorder.
- 37 percent of rapes and sexual assaults will involve offenders under the influence, and that number jumps to 90 percent when the abuses occur on college campuses.
- 15 percent of robberies, 27 percent of aggravated assaults and 25 percent of simple assaults will be carried out by individuals who've been drinking and are likely under the influence. This amounts to more than 2.5 million incidents of alcohol-related violence.
- 65 percent of intimate partner violence incidents will be carried out by perpetrators who've been drinking. This equates to more than 450,000 such incidents annually.
- 20 percent of intimate partner violence incidents involving alcohol will include the use of a gun, knife, or other potentially lethal weapons.
- 95 percent of violent crimes committed on college campuses will involve alcohol, and the total number of such assaults will be greater than 600,000.
- 118,000 incidents of family violence (spouses and partners excluded) will be linked to excessive drinking, as will 744,000 incidents of violence that involve acquaintances.
- Nearly 60 percent of violent crime victims will end up with injuries, with men being twice as likely to sustain major injuries as women.
- Overall, about 40 percent of all violent crimes will be alcohol-related.

Alcohol- Rape & Crimes

Alcohol is the #1 date rape drug. There have been over a hundred thousand drug facilitated sexual assaults and even more drug facilitated robberies per year for the last 10 years in the U.S. according to the US Department of Justice. In these cases, alcohol is used as a weapon to incapacitate the victim. The association between alcohol and rape, domestic violence, homicide and violence of all types isn't just limited to the perpetrators. Victims of these crimes are often under the influence of alcohol at the time of their victimization, their intoxication making them more vulnerable to exploitation and abuse. In the U.S. the term, slipping a "Mickey" came from a crooked bartender and his prostitute accomplices in a Chicago pub who drugged bar patrons with a solution of chloral hydrate in ethanol to rob their victims, prior to that, it was used in New York as "knock-out" drops for similar purposes. Today, the #1 way predators administer knock out drugs is through alcoholic drinks, roofies and other drugs are still used by thieves and sexual predators and if caught there is an 85% conviction rate that will land them in jail for up to 10 years where they may likely get a dose of their own medicine from other sexual predators whom they will be housed with while serving out their sentence. Based on the numbers, it is clear that alcohol abuse is a serious problem that affects many people. The general population have been subjected to ad campaigns making alcohol look fun and glamorous and the alcohol industry is slipping all drinkers a mickey, in the form of misleading ads, so to speak. The truth is alcohol renders drinkers incapacitated, many don't realize if they have been slipped a mickey or if it was just the alcohol that knocked them out. Alcohol impairs judgement and does more harm than good just like the tobacco industry we are being sold a lie and slipped a metaphorical mikey by the manufacturers with their misleading ads.

Jail Solution For Alcohol Offenses

Studies show, jail time for an addicts drug and alcohol related offenses doesn't work. Therefore, jail is not the solution for alcohol abusers related offenses with the exception of those who use alcohol as a weapon against others to commit a crime, such as in drugging and raping or robbing. Data shows that 75% of offenders who spend time in jail simply re-commit the same behaviors after jail time. At the same time, approximately 50% of all prison inmates meet criteria for substance dependence, but less than 10% receive treatment in jail. Many of these people leave prison and go right back to drinking and using. If a convicted person avoids jail to get treatment, it is mandatory to receive treatment. However, mental patients who abuse alcohol can't get better if they're not getting corrective psychological counseling and also it can only worsen the alcoholism if their getting beaten up in jail during the time they are in jail. The staff can't help if they work in fear for their safety violent inmates in addiction withdrawal. An addict in withdrawal is like a wild animal out of control. If we had programs in place to teach staff and inmates more emotional health classes and offered rehab while in jail for their alcohol addiction jail could be part of the solution. Too many violent mentally ill persons remain unmedicated in jail. On average, roughly 40 percent of inmates who are incarcerated for violent offenses were under the influence of alcohol and drugs during the time of their crime. Most people have a certain amount of self-control while sober that decreases with alcohol consumption.

Alcohol Reduces Inhibitions & Decreases Self-Control

Alcohol Lands Mental Patients In Jail Too

Those individuals with mental health issues, impulsive behavior disorders, OCD obsessive compulsive disorder or repressed anger issues are at a higher risk of making bad decisions while under the influence of alcohol. Alcohol driven offenses stem from making bad decisions while under the influence, ranging from minor to serious offenses, which includes property damage or property theft crimes, public-order offenses, disorderly conduct, assault, driving under the influence, vehicular manslaughter and homicide. Teaching inmates how to cope with repressed emotions and heal the source of their emotional and behavioral problems with mandatory mental health therapy during incarceration, could potentially be a partial-solution for the prevention of recurrence. Jail systems that provide mandatory substance abuse can intertwine with the psychiatric field of medicine with the jail providing a social worker, counseling or rehab along with a probation officer. Rehab is the only thing that will improve the outcome of those inmates who end up in the jail system multiple times for their alcohol problems. Better alcohol education is needed in jails not only for the inmates but the jail staff, as well. If you are a drinker, don't end up in jail, you may die of AWS potentially deadly alcohol withdrawal syndrome. Many have died in jail with AWS. If you work in a jail, it is in your best interest to become an expert at assessing and intervening in AWS.

Alcohol Suicide

Not all violent crimes need an attacker and a victim. Drinking alcohol is a form of self-harming behavior. According to NIH, National Institutes for Health, Suicide is an escalating public health problem and alcohol use has consistently been implicated in the precipitation of suicidal behavior. People suffering from severe depression, and who have participated in binge drinking, have a higher likelihood of experiencing suicidal thoughts and are more prone to harming themselves than people who abstain when they are depressed. Alcohol can hijack your brain and thoughts are often unreasonable thinking. According to Alcohol and Suicide Statistics. People with alcoholism are up to 120 times more likely to commit suicide than those who are not dependent on alcohol. On average, someone commits suicide every 40 seconds. 29% of suicide victims in America were found with alcohol in their system. In a sense, due to the negative health effects, over drinking and alcohol abuse is a slow form of suicide.

Accidental Death

There are many reasons to avoid drinking alcohol in excess. One of the most alarming reason is accidental death. Alcohol is a depressant and relaxant. Too much alcohol can make the drinker relax, too much, pass out and become unconscious. When a person drinks to the point of passing out, the lower esophageal sphincter (LES) that usually prevents stomach contents from entering the esophagus malfunctions as muscles relax and the sphincter may not completely close, allowing acid reflux from the stomach. Alcohol is a depressant that relaxes the body in many ways; it also relaxes the LES, allowing acid to enter the esophagus. Sadly, unexpected tragedy can strike without warning and LES can cause accidental death. Anyone who falls asleep or passed out is vulnerable to LES and asphyxiation on acid reflux. Many have died from choking on their own vomit while unconscious after passing out from drinking too much alcohol. If you have frequent heartburn or acid reflux, you are playing russian roulette by getting smashed out on alcohol. You are putting yourself at serious risk if you depend on an evening drink to help you relax. Eventually, the risk becomes more dangerous. The safest solution is to quit drinking and try replacing alcohol with chamomile or hemp herbal tea. The herbs safely relax you without any know risk as associated with alcohol. Drink caffeine free herbal teas rather than alcohol right before bed for relaxing sleep.

Alcohol Murders

According to a domestic violence study 90% of the time, the best predictor of domestic violence is past behavior and substance abuse. According to a US Department of Justice study, Most murders inside the family happen at night (62%) and Alcohol was often part of the fatal scenario. Nearly 1/2 of the killers and 1/3 of their victims had been drinking at the time of the family homicide. The remaining majority had some type of mental issue and 100% of murderers have poor anger management and relationship skills. Intimate partner violence had previously occurred in 70% of them. Interestingly, only 25% of prior domestic violence appeared in the arrest records. Additionally, according to researchers at John Hopkins, a study titled, "Men Who Murder Their Families" revealed,"The most common type of killer was a possessively jealous type and many of the men who commit murder-suicide, as well as those who kill their children, also seem to fit that profile." "A jealous substance abuser with a gun poses a particularly deadly combination of factors; one that was present in about 40 percent of the killers." Additionally, over enmeshment is a condition in which they view "their" family members as "possessions" that they "control" or they don't see any boundaries between their identity, their wife's identity or their children's individual identities. The murderer views the killings as part of his suicide, a familyside of the entire family, where the anomic, overly enmeshed individual can't bear to leave the pain behind and so he takes his wife and children with him". Prevention's National Violent Death Reporting System statistics show in most homicide- suicide cases, the perpetrators were men (91 %) and most used a gun (88%).

Jail Alcohol- Homebrew

The prison alcohol industry probably started flourishing about a week after history's first alcohol dependant prisoner was incarcerated. Alcohol makers risk getting in trouble with jailers and risk doing even more jail time if caught making homebrew alcohol while in jail. However, many inmates are so dependant on self-medicating with alcohol, that even after they are incarcerated, they will still go to extremes to get an alcohol buzz after being sentenced and are serving their jail time. Still making jail alcohol is a risk some are willing to take. It is illegal and jailers will confiscate it if they find it. The inmates who make jail alcohol, have very few commodities they can use as leverage in commerce and they are willing to take necessary risk to have jail alcohol to sell or trade and rack up other inmate indebtedness to have a sense of power and control within the system. Even though it is illegal, homemade jail Alcohol is a hot commodity that is boot-legged in jail. It is traded amongst inmates for goodies and necessities such as cookies, socks, deodorant, tissue ect. Their have been instances where prison brew masters or boot leggers have even killed fellow inmates for unpaid debt racked up for alcohol. Alcohol in prison is controlled by gangs or basically the prison mob control the making and distribution and trade of jail alcohol. Homemade prison alcohol goes by a multitude of names, including juice, jump, raisin jack, brew, hooch, and pruno made from prunes. Pruno has been the source of many deaths due to botulism. Jail house wine is derived by mixing rotting fruit with sugar, water and heating it in the sink hiding in warm, unsanitary places within the prison. Botulinum produces the deadliest toxin known to humans, it is 6 million times deadlier than rattlesnake venom. In jail they make alcoholic beverages a plastic garbage bag with rotten fruit, sugar, yeast, soda and a kicker and keep it hot for several days burping the bag until it ferments. This method is high risk for producing botulism. Many inmates have fallen ill, been hospitalized and died from drinking prison alcohol. Some of the symptoms of botulism are:

- Double vision
- Blurred vision
- Drooping eyelids
- Slurred speech
- Difficulty swallowing
- A thick-feeling tongue
- Dry mouth
- Muscle weakness

As botulism poisoning gets worse, more symptoms develop, such as:

- Dehydration
- Difficulty breathing
- Paralysis (can't move your body)
- Death

Firefighters, Medics, and Law Enforcement Have High Use Rates

Our super heros are human, too. As compared to the general public, there are higher rates of on the job trauma and post traumatic stress leading to mental illness, psychological trauma, including substance abuse, addiction, and suicide amongst our police and emergency professionals. According to the Bureau of Labor Statistics, there are approximately 806,400 people who serve as police officers, detectives, and game wardens. The majority of these officers, self-medicate and many use alcohol, too. According to Substance Abuse and Mental Health Services Administration reports, about one in five adults or 43.8 million Americans in the United States was living with a diagnosable mental health disorder in 2013. Additionally, they found that about 9.3 million Americans considered taking their own lives that year. First responders, including law enforcement and firefighters, are certainly part of this statistic but many feel they have to be tough, feel they can't talk about their job stress and trauma and end up self-medicating which can lead to addiction for them, too.

Police are among the professions with the highest rates of alcohol use. Researchers with the "Badge of Life" program, point out that stress and depression is high amongst officers and 126 police officers committed suicide in 2012 alone. In 2018, more police died of suicide than in the line of duty. The average age of suicidal officers was 42 and the average time on the job was 16 years. These officers were beaten down by years of hard work dealing with dangerous criminals and poor coping skills which has lead many officers to self-medicating, after work, with alcohol and other substances. Many sustain injuries performing very physical job duties and self-medicate their own physical and mental pain. Additionally, officers are under constant mental pressure to obey the law themselves or lose their jobs. According to police crisis organization, "Blue H.E.L.P" at least 159 officers took their own lives in 2018, in the United States. The same number of officer suicides were tracked in 2017. Remember to thank our officers for doing the job of keeping themselves and us all safe. Clearly, jail is not the best place for self-medicating alcoholics to get better.

The Tragic Truth Of Alcohol Abuse

Alcohol abuse is now a national epidemic and great numbers of people are dying from it. It is even affecting our criminal justice system workers all the way up to our nation's leaders in the white house. A flash-mob of people are dying daily from the negative health effects of alcohol. Over 88,000 people died in the U.S. from alcohol related deaths last year. 8,000 to 10,000 of these alcohol deaths were underaged kids. Alcohol kills more people each year than all other drug overdoses.

Alcohol is the 3rd Leading Cause of Preventable Death in the United States.

In addition, Alcohol drinkers also die of co-morbid diseases and disorders associated with alcohol abuse such as; cirrhosis of the liver, fatty liver disease, various cancers, pancreatitis, organ failure, suicide, DTs withdraw and other alcohol impaired accident related deaths.

Death Toll Drunk Driving

Alcohol-impaired driving accounts for more than 30 % of all driving fatalities each year. Drunk drivers account for 70% of driving fatalities, where there is a known alcohol-test result for the driver but it is likely that the percentage is even higher.

HOLIDAY ALCOHOL RELATED FATAL TRAFFIC ACCIDENTS

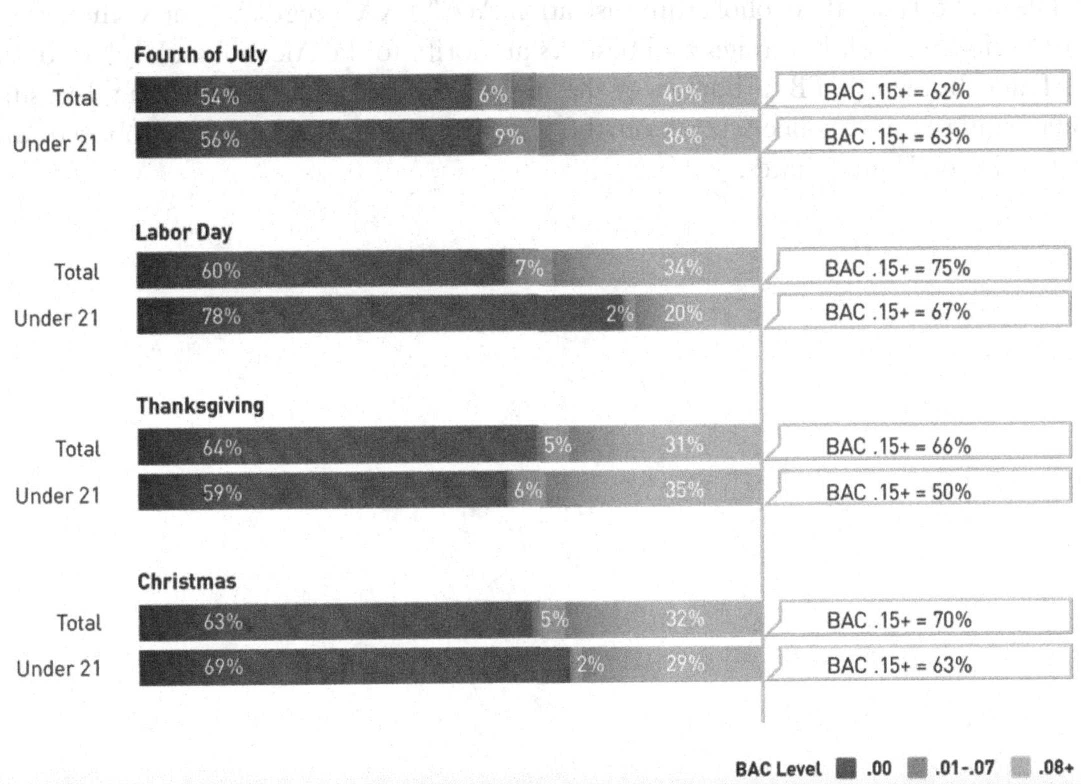

This chart, courtesy of the National Highway Traffic Safety Administration, indicates alcohol related holiday death rates and 37,133 people died in traffic crashes in 2017 in the United States and 68% of those were in crashes that at least one driver in the crash had a BAC of .15 or higher, which is almost double the legal limit of 0.08% or less.

How Alcohol Abuse Became An Epidemic

Americans are self medicating their pain. There is a pain epidemic. There is an Opiate epidemic and there is an Alcohol epidemic. Apparently, the public service announcements have not been adequate. Awareness is the first step to solve any problem and awareness is the first step to quit any bad habit. It is our own individual responsibility to educate ourselves and our families until government public health systems can adequately address America's drinking problem and provide better educational awareness campaigns to all communities.

Who Regulates Alcohol

Surprisingly, The Food and Drug Administration does not regulate alcoholic beverages. The FDA regulates all dietary consumable products and also the labels on liquids such as red wine vinegar and non-alcoholic beer but the FDA not regulate alcohol, that is why we see the government warnings on alcohol but usually don't see a nutritional facts label on alcohol, currently, they only regulate the labeling of some wine and beer. The Federal Alcohol Administration Act ("FAA") regulates the commerce of wine, spirits and malt beverages and bestows authority to the Alcohol and Tobacco Tax and Trade Bureau (TTB) a bureau of the United States Department of the Treasury, which regulates and collects taxes on the trade and import of alcohol, tobacco, and firearms in the United States.

Chapter 6

Who Is To Blame? The Psychology & Genetics Of Alcohol Addiction

Because of the sugar content, Alcohol is more addictive than any other drug as it blocks more neurotransmitters than any other drug. All drugs of abuse, including alcohol, act on our brain's feel good reward system, the system that transfers neurotransmitter signals and primarily dopamine. The function of the neurotransmitter system is affected by environmental and genetic factors. One of those genetic factors is HK2 which is an RNA virus that integrates within a gene to regulate the activity of dopamine. The HK2 integration is most commonly found in people with substance use disorders, and individuals with the HK2 genetic factor will usually have a proclivity for addiction. However, drinking alcohol is a freedom of choice, so the decision to drink alcohol is on the individual. Every drinker, makes the choice to do so. It would be a good idea to have a HK2 genome test to know your risk. There is always the psychological aspect to addiction and alcoholism. Exposure to an alcoholic role-model has proven to be a factor in research studies. Many emotional factors drive our behaviors must be taken into account. Additionally, genetic factors play a role as well. You can take a DNA test to see if you have the addiction gene. As much as 60% of alcoholics have a genetic inheritance of addiction or alcoholism traits, which meaning they inherited an alcoholic vulnerability from either a parent, a grandparent or both, regardless of environmental influences. So, with that gene you could blame your parents ancestral line. When it comes to psychology, according to Freudian psychology, we say one thing and we mean our mother, not exactly, but hopefully you get the picture. Children are a blank slate at birth and soak up information like sponges as they learn and grow. While it is true that early childhood conditioning to substance abuse is a factor, I do not believe the philosophy that everything is your mother's fault. Mom's can be distracted from their babies from being stressed by living with abusive fathers and older children are equally influenced by other caregivers, such as older siblings, babysitters and early childhood teachers. Attachment issues can lead to alcoholism in adulthood. The alcohol gene theory has almost been disproven, but setting an alcohol use example to your children is a trait that can be inherited from either parent can cause an increased non-genetic risk. Not enough unconditional love throughout life can be a risk factor. We must take into account the roles of other primary caregivers in the early developmental and most impressionable stages of life. If a person has an alcoholic parent or primary caregiver, in early childhood it is considered predisposition and increased risk factor for alcohol abuse as an adult, also. There are some studies linking it to not getting our needs met as babies, developing unhealthy coping and relationship skills thereafter and self medicating to suppress emotional pain of not ever getting our needs met.

Love is the drug we have all been looking for!

Adult Pacifier or Bottle Comfort & Attachment Disorders

According to recent studies, life is full of challenges and difficulties and the more traumatic events we experience as a child may bear a factor in a person's proclivity to use alcohol to try to self medicate our unresolved emotional injuries and issues. A baby sucks a pacifier to calm and soothe its cries, an adult may suck down a bottle of alcohol to calm and ease themself but at some point the bottle sucks the life out of the person. There is no lasting nourishment in alcohol and it is a depressant. Alcohol is not a good substance of choice for lasting feel good solution. Cultivating meaningful relationships and life experiences and by finding joy in the simple things in life is a source of true and lasting peace and happiness that you will never get from a bottle.

However, it is a fact that many alcoholic men and women are found to have undergone early attachment trauma during important childhood developmental stages, resulting in interpersonal difficulties later on in life that may have made them more susceptible to alcohol and drug abuse.

In fact, having a father that is an alcoholic and a mother suffering from obsessive compulsive disorder (OCD) is considered a background that provides fertile grounds for an addiction. It also poses difficulties in the person being able to develop secure and intimate attachments with others as often their emotional needs were ignored by the alcoholic parent(s) therefore they never were nurtured to develop good coping skills having had alcoholic roll models.

According to the CDC and NIH studies, there is some link to addiction and attachment disorders and therefore in those cases, professional psychological care is needed as part of recovery. Additionally, as a part of self-care in recovery and sobriety it is good to talk to a professional counselor, work on healing childhood wounds and read books on childhood development and some shadow work as part of an integrative recovery process.

Glamorized & Glorified Alcohol Industry Marketing

How did our culture get here? Alcohol is a drug. We've all been taught about the dangers of drugs, and perhaps overlook that alcohol is in fact a drug. Alcohol is a big industry. We are merely consumers to the Alcohol giants. Corporations only care about their bottom line profits. The problems that alcohol creates in people's lives are of no concerns of its producers, it's strictly business to them and they are out for one thing only, to make money. All the industry cares about you is to make money from your purchase of alcohol. Its a cat and mouse game, they make the alcohol and cleverly attractive ads, you buy the product and chi ching ching, they have your money in the bank and doesnt matter at all to them if you eventually end up on skid row. Many alcohol based herbal remedies that were intended to be administered in a single ½ ounce dose have been marketed as one of the latest drink sensation, for example a popular german digestive aid and cough suppressant that was kept in nearly every german grandma's medicine cabinet for centuries became the biggest seller in U.S. nightclubs by mixing it with an energy drink sort of like the old car-bomb drink concept. There was a massive marketing campaign directed toward U.S. millenial party-goers as the latest rave drink and instantly became the world's best-selling liqueur brand. The popular stomach digestive medicine was never intended to be consumed by binge-drinking teens and people died from consuming too much of the digestive aid with energy drinks, creating alcohol overdose complicated by caffeine overdose, which may cause life threatening heart complications and heart failure. The alcohol industry is responsible for their ad campaigns just as the tobacco industry touted cigarettes as being good for health. Alcohol is dangerous to your health. Beware of clever marketing.

Lead Us Not Into Temptation

The Alcohol industry mandates that manufacturers put a disclaimer warning label on each bottle of their product leaving it up to the consumer to accept full responsibility for their own health and safety while under the influence of their product. The beverage industry is heavily dependent on you for their profits. Alcohol advertisement campaign spending has increased 400% in the last forty years. In 1999, the alcohol industry spent two billion dollars annually per year on all media advertising according to the Strasburger report. The beer brewing industry itself spent more than $770 million on television ads and $15 million on radio ads in 2000 according to the Center for Science in the Public Interest.

Alcohol Advertising Fueling The Fire

The alcohol industry spend billions in ad campaigns, yearly, to entice you to drink and at the end of every televised commercials they simply state, "Drink Responsibly." We have not adequately been educated about the dangers of alcohol. One of the main reasons is money, is the heaviest drinkers are of greatly disproportionate importance to the sales and profitability of the alcoholic-beverage industry. "If the top drinkers somehow could be induced to curb their consumption level to that of the next lower group, then total ethanol sales would fall by 60 %." In other words, if alcoholics quit drinking the alcohol industry sales would fall by 60 %. Alcohol suppliers said sales were at $25.2 billion in 2017 in the United States, according to the Distilled Spirits Council.

In a 2015 study, state and local governments collected $16 billion from alcohol taxes, they have collected much more since then.

Homebrew Alcohol Use

One of the most well-known homebrew beer recipes was from the United States' first president George Washington's "Small" Beer. While serving in the Virginia militia prior to his presidency, Washington recorded his now-infamous small beer recipe in his diary which is now in possession of the New York Public Library. Making homemade spirits has long been a part of American culture, albeit it was often illegal in most states. Homebrewing was federally legalized in 1978 for the first time since Prohibition made it illegal in 1919. However, regulation of alcohol is predominantly left to the states. In 2013, Mississippi and Alabama, the last two states remaining with laws against homebrewing, passed legislation to permit beer brewing at home. Today, there are currently 1.1 million people in the United States who homebrew their own beer. Many of these are healthier than commercially manufactured because they contain less chemicals in the processing. Only small doses can be considered safe but it is important to look at the magnatured of homebrewing as it is not included in many of the alcohol sales statistics studies. However, American Homebrewers Association recent survey shows:

- In 2017, homebrewer's will have produced more than 1.4 million barrels of brew representing 1% of total U.S. production.
- Homebrewers are spread across the country, with 31% in the South, 26% in the Midwest, 24% in the Northeast and 19% in the West.
- The average homebrewer is 42 years old and 52% are between ages 30-49.
- 85 % are married or in a domestic partnership.
- 68 % have a college degree or some form of higher education, and nearly 68% have household incomes of $75,000 or more

We have no idea of what the associated health impacts are of homebrew consumption or how it affects the families who consume it, however, high levels of acetaldehyde found in homemade liquor, beer and wine, which may likely be due to improper production and brewing methods that may lead to an increase in the bacteria that increases the level of acetaldehyde.

Alcohol Deaths

The Centers for Disease Control (CDC) reported that there are more than 19,000 annual deaths due to alcoholic liver disease and more than 30,000 people die from alcohol-induced deaths from accidents, homicides or other incidents. Alcoholism is a problem, and the statistics couldn't be clearer. Educating people about alcoholism, functional alcoholism and alcohol abuse is the first step in making a change.

There are many organizations that provide free information to bring awareness to the alcohol problem as a public health issue. There are community awareness programs and those who are successful at quitting are valued to share their story with others in the community to raise awareness. There are many organizations who care about saving lives and preventing alcohol related traffic accidents through education at responsibility.org, their efforts have saved many lives over the last decade.

In 2017, the rate of alcohol-impaired driving fatalities per 100,000 population was 3.4, representing a 63% decrease since 1982, when record-keeping began, and a 46% decrease since the inception of The Foundation for Advancing Alcohol Responsibility in 1991. Still, more than 15 million people struggle with an alcohol use disorder in the United States, which means less people are driving while intoxicated with alcohol. Less than 8% of the 15 million with alcohol use disorder receive treatment.

According to the Centers for Disease Control, 6-8 people die every day from drinking alcohol too quickly, this is known as alcohol poisoning. The number one way college students who die from beer-bonging is from alcohol poisoning, that is simply the result of drinking too much alcohol too quickly. About 76% of the people who die are men. Most alcoholics die from liver disease, cirrhosis and alcoholic hepatitis. This is a horribly unpleasant way to die and an alcoholic who takes Acetaminophen with alcohol still in their system can cause kidney disease and failure.

Ignition Interlocks

According to Mothers-Against-Drunk-Driving (MADD) in-car breathalyzers, force prior offenders to provide a sober breath sample before operating their vehicles. MADD has successfully pushed for laws requiring these devices for drunk driving offenders in 30 states. According to the research, if ignition interlocks were adopted nationwide, an additional 1,000 lives could be saved each year. It would be great if the government made it a standard on all new car manufacturing that would cut drunk driving to zero.

Most Drinkers Have An Early History With Alcohol

Alcohol kills more teenagers than all other drugs combined. It is a factor in the three leading causes of death among 15- to 24-year-olds: accidents, homicides and alcohol related death. Studies show that many of the teens had one or both parents or a primary caregiver who were also alcohol users.

Everyone Has An Alcohol Story

We each have our own story of when alcohol was introduced into our lives and during recovery it is important to share your story in a supportive environment. I too, have experienced some devastating alcohol tragedies throughout my life and with 70% of the adult population having had alcohol this year, we all have a story regarding alcohol.

What is yours? I could tell you about when I was a child and my friend and I were kidnapped and terrorized by a bunch of drunk rednecks. Needless, to say, I was totally turned off from the effects of alcohol on other people's behavior from the first time I ever saw it being abused. After witnessing a few despicable drunken scenarios throughout my life, I never thought that I could have a problem with alcohol use. I was raised better. My mom never drank or smoked, neither did any of her female siblings, my grandmother on my father's side, was from the prohibition era and she said her generation believed it wasnt lady-like and therefore, it was strictly forbidden in my grandma Peters and my mother's homes. However, I was aware my grandfather, my father, uncles, several cousins (on both sides) and my older siblings and myself were individually, having drinks away from home.

My first awareness of drinking, that I remember, was at my mom's father's house, my grandfather. He had a cool Hawaiian hula-dancer tattoo on his forearm from his days in the navy, he was light hearted, played the harmonica and as far back as I can remember, he was a country doctor of sorts that made herbal plant medicines. Mom said that he learned it from one of our great grandmothers who was an Indian medicine woman. Mom said people would line up around the house, with their babies for grandpa to treat them and their babies for colic and he made medicinal poultice for the pain of breast feeding mothers. Grandpa was amazing, he made many remedies and one medicine that cured a skin rash that I had, virtually overnight and he also was a winemaker. I was amazed by Grandpa and he always had a garden, a small orchard and vineyard. My grandma on my dad's side also, had a garden and she grew many of her own foods too and made homemade milk products such as butter. Once, when I was about 5 years old, grandpa was making red wine and sampling it and I asked, him if I could taste it, too. He laughed and gave me a taste which I remember making a facial expression that made him laugh. It was a face like when a baby bites into a lemon, it was intense. After that, I remember, I was a hyper child and it was hard for my grandparents to watch me, I was always running off to the neighbors house or climbing up in trees, sometimes they would give me things to calm me down so I wouldn't be so hyperactive. I remember grandpa would give me a small amount of wine or coffee which have the opposite effect on a child, and makes them slow down or sleep. Several times throughout childhood I remember taking sips of his wine. You may think, it is wrong to give children alcohol, yes! However, this is nothing uncommon many cultures, including in the U.S, have been known to give sick or fussy children alcohol.

Giving Children Alcohol

Many children's teething medicines and cough medicines contain alcohol. When you give your child these common over the counter medicines, you are in fact giving them alcohol. For centuries, people have been giving children alcohol based medicines and some even gave their children a thimble of rum and other alcohol for teething pain for centuries. Today, this will land you in jail and your children in custody of child protective services and foster care followed by extensive family counseling to get them back.

My Early Childhood Alcohol Experience

When I was 3-4 years old I overdosed on child fever liquid and baby aspirins and had to have my stomach pumped. When I was 5 or 6, I overdosed on children's cough syrup and again, had to have my stomach pumped. Child medicines are filled with sugar to make the alcohol based medicines taste better. I am not sure if was something environmental or genetic that I may have been born with or if I learned by exposure but also, I remember that on my dad's side of the family we had some uncles that heavily abused alcohol and one that dad kept at a safe distance from us, because everyone in the family was afraid of him when he would drink because he could become quite violent when he was drinking. My dad, was the kind of person who had a lot of friends, my mom always said he never met a stranger and he was the kind of guy that would give you the shirt of his back. Dad would lend a helping hand to strangers and neighbors, he would stop and help a stranger if their car was broken down and he was ex-military. Dad did drink but not in the household or in front of us younger children out of respect for my mom and being a good fatherly role model. I only remember once at age 10, seeing dad drink and it was at one of my dad's friends house, my dad had a glass of orange juice and I asked for a drink of it and he said, no, that he was drinking grown up orange juice. He did not let me taste it.

Two of my older sisters had married and left the home when I was 7- 9 years old and one lived in another state and the other lived in europe then when I was 10 years old, my father tragically died in an automobile accident, in the late 70's my newly widowed mom worked night shift to support the remaining family and I remember my older brother always having to babysit me and my younger sister, he was only 17 and understandably he seemed upset often and avoided communication as much as possible with me as I was also, an especially very inquisitive child. I am sure he had stress from being parentatized acting as a surrogate father as a teen and would have probably preferred hanging out with his football team buddies. My brother was the quarterback of our high school football team and most popular guy in our town but also he had been my male role model since dad died. It was the late 70's all american culture and I remember him having a couple of high school parties at our house when mom was working night shift and all the teenagers were laughing and having a good time, they were cool, they listened to cool music and would drink, just like a typical teenage party. I was 12 years old, so his solution for not corrupting us was to lock me and my younger sister up in the back bedroom and we were not allowed to come out, that was the rule. I was curious and scared because I could smell smoke and where there is smoke there is fire. In those days, people would have bonfires. During harvest festivals and football season. I would peak out the windows and one of my brothers friends caught me spying and came into my room and gave me sips of his beer. Also, he was cute, flirty and super drunk, I was pouting because I was locked in a bedroom and couldn't come out to the party, he shared his beer with me and said when you grow up you can be my girlfriend. It felt good to have someone to talk to me, to be nice, to not treat me like a burden and to give me attention and he was a really cute teenager, too. I thought when I grow up, I'll have friends to talk to and I'll drink beer just like him and be a cool teenager. From that point forward, I associated drinking with being a cool grown-up. I could not wait to grow up. My brother was strict, he made sure we did our chores and for his young age, he was a good protector and made sure no harm came to us.

In the late 70's America was a party culture the only real deterrent I had as a teen growing up was the influence of my mom and her zero tolerance for drinking, her generation of women had a strict no-drinking rule and her grandparents generation were from the pre-great depression era during prohibition when there was a total ban on alcohol. In my generation X, lots of girls and women were drinking alcohol. I was a majorette and the school imposed a code-of-conduct, sort of code-of-honor, it was against the rules for misconduct in uniform and I didnt want to risk getting kicked off the majorette squad.

According to alcohol research and statistics, my early childhood exposures increase my risk of alcohol abuse as an adult. However, after a person is educated and becomes aware, a person can't blame their childhood experiences, conditioning, parents, peers or siblings. When every drinker decides to drink, its their own individual choice. Most of my caregivers no longer drink alcohol, either.

Parenting- Men Vrs. Women- Dad Vs Mom- Alcohol Consumption

Statistically, Men have alcohol use disorder twice as often as women. In a 2012 study, of the 17 million adults with alcohol use disorder 11.2 million were men and 5.7 million were women. Parents may not like to think about it but the truth is that many kids and teens try alcohol before it is legal for them to drink it. As a parent, even if you proclaim a negative attitude toward liquor and you have it in the household, your child will think twice about using alcohol but will likely drink your alcohol when your away. If you are a heavy drinker, your child is 3 x more likely to drink, also. When it comes to alcohol, children follow their parents example more often than not.

Childhood Drinkers

Usually have an adult supplier. When caregivers give alcohol to children, those children are three times more likely to binge drink as adults. There are several ways minors get alcohol and they're all fairly easy but they're all illegal. Almost 72 percent of teens who drink get alcohol without having to pay for it and 45% of them are high school girls. Many kids simply take it from their parents alcohol stores, when their not looking. It is estimated that 855,000 underaged youth between 12-17 years of age have an alcohol use disorder. It is a crime to give children alcohol and adults can be charged with a criminal misdemeanor or a felony for supplying alcohol to minors under U.S. law.

Teachers and Alcohol Abuse

In our culture, teachers are expected to be a good example to their students by being teetotalers, but statistically, it's not that way. Teachers are among the highest stressed professionals. By most measures, teachers are the most stressed and most underpaid, undervalued, and underappreciated workers in America today. The reality is substance abuse and addiction levels are high in the education industry, many use alcohol to cope with their high stress. It is a domino effect, and students are affected by their teachers stress management. Teachers who went to a college or university that had a strong culture of heavy alcohol consumption is an added influential factor. The stress of the education industry may also exacerbate pre-existing mental health conditions, including substance use disorders. In the study, 80 percent said they felt stressed while they were at work; 70 percent further said that their work left them feeling exhausted, and 66 percent said they had difficulty sleeping because of the strain of teaching. Teachers are among the professions with the highest rates of alcoholism.

The Effect Of Alcohol On Young Adult Lives

After high-school, every young adult makes some serious coming of age decisions. Many young adults start out life in college. Many do not choose to go to college, immediately. All young adults are faced with decisions that will shape their future and their life path. Researchers estimate that each year:

- Research shows that young adults age 18-25 have a stronger proclivity for impulsive behaviors, but that decreases after age 25.
- 1,825 college students between the ages of 18 and 24 die from alcohol-related unintentional injuries, including motor-vehicle crashes.
- 696,000 students, ages 18 to 24 were assaulted by other students who had been drinking.
- Many of these face legal issues from the consequences of behavior under the influence of alcohol
- Poor decisions are made while under the influence of alcohol.
- A new drinker never knows how alcohol is going to affect their behavior.

It is clear that alcohol has the potential of ruining young lives. All young adults with make a decision at some point to become a drinker or non-drinker. Drinking alcohol is a personal decision each person makes to drink alcohol or to abstain and that is the individual's choice. Psychology changes as society changes and evolves and the old cookie-cutter means of summing people up and putting them in a psychological box, is no longer valid.

Just like a coming of age party that involves alcohol. When people turn 21, most young adults in America celebrate that birthday by legally drinking alcohol for the first time.

21st Birthday Is Not A Coming of Drinking Age Party

Turning 21 is a coming of legal adult age party but has been massively marketed as a right of passage to legally drink alcohol, in America. It is important to make sure the young adults in your life are presented with other options of celebrating without making alcohol a part of their turning 21 birthday party. Turning 21 means you are a full grown adult.

How Alcohol Affected My Late Teen Young Adult Life

I was one of those teens that tried beer with my girlfriends and cousins. Just like many teens across America, we would sneak to get beer after school but luckily I hated the taste. I had a part time job when I was 15 and I met my first boyfriend. He was 19 and he had big dreams. I was always a talker and I finally had someone I could talk my head off to. I had big dreams of being a college majorette and becoming a fashion designer making flashy costumes for performers. He wanted to be a doctor, a chiropractor and help people because he had kyphosis and painful back problems growing up. He wanted to travel and live the American dream. When he was a child, his father was a preacher and I saw the photos of him at his baptism. He was a christian, he came from a good family, well respected in the community. From the outside looking in, his family was the kind of family all parents would want their daughter marrying into. His dad was the president of the local masons lodge and they did philanthropy fund raisers for the shriners and children's hospitals. After graduation, he asked me to be his girl, gave me a nice diamond ring and promised me the most wonderful life. We had a life plan and it sounded so good that I chose to turn down my full scholarship to the top university in the state and marry my best friend and high school sweetheart. I was 18 and he was 22. We were young and in love and had an exciting dream of being free from our parents and starting our own family. I was so happy, I thought I was finally going to have a big happy family. We planned to build a big house and living happily ever after, but sometimes life takes unexpected twist and turns, especially when alcohol dependency is involved.

Alcohol Home Invasion

Alcohol can come crashing down your door and invade the lives of your loved ones, unexpectedly, much like a home invasion. As an adult, I still did not like the taste of beer or mixed drinks but my husband, loved it! Once he got a taste, he could never get enough and he didn't know when to stop. All the friends that he had were drinkers, and all of their wives were drinkers, too. We had a dinner party with one of the managers from his work, whose wife brought a bottle of wine and she was a wine drinker. I became friends with her and began to casually drink a little wine with her on the weekends at our dinner parties. Soon my husband was invited to go through initiation ceremonies to become a mason. We began going to VFW, Masons and Elks lodge parties, he had hurt his back lifting boxes of produce at work was drinking more and more and self-medicating his pain with alcohol. I did not realize his drinking was getting out of hand. We did not drink at all during the work-week, only socially on the weekend. At that stage, I didn't really like or enjoy it, either. I did it to fit in with the people in my husbands family and his social group of friends. I didn't give his drinking much thought at that stage, as we were both working hard to make money and bought our first property with a beautiful creek and babbling brook running through it, just outside the city limits and I took a drafting class and drew our own blueprints. We custom designed our house plans.

He was making a good living as a department manager so he decided to make a career of it and gave up on his dream of becoming a chiropractor. We just bought land and were planning to build our first house, so we would have had to move to another state for several years to go to a chiropractic college. I believe this was a source of disappointment in his life but alcohol killed his motivation. He had many secret issues that he would brood over when he would drink. I could see some things were coming to a head inside of him and even though I tried to help him, alcohol affected his brain in a way that he was becoming more and more combative. I tried to help him "snap out of it" with love. I tried to set an example by becoming totally focused on starting our family and I was pregnant with our daughter. Nothing, I could say or do seemed to help. Nothing, I did to fix the problem would change anything, he was in the grips of alcohol. His supervisors were putting a lot of stress on him to meet quotas. The more stress the job put on him, the more he began to drink and get frustrated. I began to realize he was drinking way too much, he would drink 1/5 of whiskey in a night. He had a lot of emotions he wasn't dealing with inside and when he would drink too much his anger issues would come out and he would take it out on me.

Alcohol Depletes Serotonin in the Brain Causing Aggression In Some Drinkers

At the time, I didn't understand the science of alcohol dependance or the effects it has on brain chemistry. I tried to fix the problem with words. I encouraged him to deal with his back pain through chiropractic and talk out his feelings and cut back on his drinking. At the time I didn't understand how addiction grabs a person and it changes their personality uncontrollably. The more I tried to talk him out of drinking, the more he drank and the worse our relationship became. I was sucked into his world and codependent. I wanted to help him and thought I could fix him. At one point I even got a job at a doctors office so he would have constant access to chiropractic care for his back pain. When he was only 23, I realized that he had something in him that had such a powerful control over him that he could not control it himself. He had deep repressed emotional pain and I could see that he was self medicating with alcohol and it was causing big problems between us. Additionally, he wasn't handling the stress of adulthood responsibilities very well. I was beginning to see some type of mental illness emerging, triggered by the alcohol. I watched his brain chemistry change him into a different person, that I didn't know anymore. Our arguments where compounded by the fact that we had very different views on substance use and abuse, he felt normal with drugs and alcohol as a means of self-medicating due to his family history.

Alcohol Induced Serotonin Deficient

When alcohol enters the bloodstream, it also affects the nervous system and brain cells and cause brain functions to produce more neurotransmitters such as serotonin and dopamine. When a large amount of alcohol is consumed, high levels of serotonin can be produced, and normal behaviour is impaired. Overuse and abuse of alcohol over time causes a serotonin deficit in the brain. Because serotonin has such an effect on the body and the brain, a lack of serotonin in the body can lead to some unpleasant symptoms. These include:

- Anger and irritable
- digestive problems (including heartburn and constipation)
- Aches and an increased sensitivity to pain
- odd eating patterns (including binge eating carbohydrates)
- separation anxiety
- dependency
- sleep schedules
- Low self-esteem
- headaches and migraines
- bad moods
- putting the blame for their "problem" on others

Brain-Derived Neurotrophic Factor (BDNF) in Alcoholism

Alcohol may be particularly damaging to key components of the "brain reward system." Alcohol sensitizes dopamine and serotonin neurons to toxic excessive excitation also known as excitotoxicity. The brain growth hormone called brain-derived neurotrophic factor BDNF, can help protect neurons against excitotoxicity. BDNF is a protein that, in humans, is encoded by the BDNF Gene. BDNF is a member of the neurotrophin family of growth factors, which are related to nerve growth factor. Neurotrophic factors are found in the brain and in the peripheral nervous system pathways. Studies suggests that BDNF synthesis determine success at long-term sobriety and abstinence.

Abusive Mind Games & Bullying

If you are living with someone with alcoholism or addiction expect them to deny they have a problem, denial is part of the alcoholism disease process. Expect them to try to blame you in some way for their drinking, but, don't let yourself be bullied or pulled into the addict's world. It is their choice to drink and if they are alcohol dependant, they are beyond it being a simple choice, if they are dependant, they feel they need to drink alcohol to feel normal. The more you try to take measures to encourage or force them to stop drinking, the angrier they will become with you. If you are threatened, verbally abused or manipulated seek professional help or support and you may even have to distance yourself if you are physically abused or endangered, it is necessary to have them picked up on a 5150 psychiatric well care evaluation for proper rehabilitation. Although your support is crucial for a loved one's recovery, do not let yourself be pulled into the addict's illogical world or tolerate abuse. Your mental health is important. Addicts will try to play mind games when you no longer feel sorry for them and when you stop enabling them. They will often try to blame you and make you feel guilty in some way for their problem. It is not your fault, however, mentally impaired people tend to blame and take it out on the present person closest to them. If you feel threatened, used, manipulated or otherwise endangered in their presence, seek legal or professional counseling and distance yourself until you can re-engage safely and respectfully.

Dwindling Relationship WIth An Alcoholic

In reality, all of our problems stemmed from alcohol, but when I was living through it, I thought we just had different feelings when it came to family structure and values. He was an only child, I was the 4th of 5 children and very use to a large family lifestyle. He was raised that drinking in the home was acceptable, I was not. I wanted at least 3 children, a clean family home environment, a couple of dogs and cats. The more mature I became with age, the more immature he seemed to become with alcohol. Once alcohol took over his life, that is all he wanted to do, and to drink freely in his home. I am not sure of all the things he was dealing with or the other substances he may have been using secretively, it was always his defense to blame his behavior on the alcohol. The more independent I became the more we grew apart. An alcoholic spouse often resents their spouse as they become dependant on them. We spend our childhood trying to gain our independence from our parents because we all want to have our freedom to be ourselves and live on our own as adults, often we chose partners with the same problems we never resolved with our parents so we have the chance to heal the issues with our parents through our partners, which is totally illogical and only causes resentment between couples. That is why it is important to work through your inner child wounds before you marry. When we don't work on healthing our emotional wounds we bring the scars of them into our relationship and it causes marital problems. As for our situation, turns out, we were raised with a totally different view of substance use, also. On my side, I had the influence of my mom whom did not believe in taking any medications, except in emergencies. While on his side of the family they were all drinkers, on the other side of his family they viewed prescription drugs as medicine and all of the women were taking nerve pills. His grandmother was a surgical nurse and another cousin was also a nurse. This was the source of his early introduction to alcohol use.

Nurses Medical Workers And Alcohol

Nurses are extremely important in providing healthcare to patients. Working in medical healthcare can be a stress filled career path. Sadly, nurses commit suicide at a higher rate than any other healthcare professional and are 4 times more likely to commit suicide than people outside the medical field.

Dependence on Alcohol and Drugs Among Nurses is around 10% of all Nurses.

There are around 4 million nurses in America, that is 4 times the number of physicians. Nurses sometimes work 12 hour shifts, they report suffering from exhaustion more than other workers, they go from one emotionally and physically demanding patient emergency or crisis to another with little time to destress. People in nursing and other helping professions show higher rates of alcohol addiction than in other lines of work. About 83 % of healthcare professionals consumed alcohol in the last year. About 80 % of nurses with an alcohol use disorder have an alcoholic family member. According to studies, nurses have a higher tendency as enablers and may ignore colleagues displaying signs of abuse or cover up signs of alcoholism in themselves. The study revealed that many of the nurses polled, view drinking in excess as normal behavior based on their job pressures and family history.

Chapter 7

Our Alcohol Related Family History

Aside from the nurses in our family, I also soon realized that every female on his side of the family and many on my side of the family, had emotional problems and were dependant on sedative or tranquilizer type prescription medications. His side of our family had the belief that if you felt some intense emotions to take a pill and chill, on my side, it was the silent pink elephant in the room. Even more alarming, was when I found out his family had been medicating my husband with their own adult prescription medications, since he was a child. Once we got into a spat and his mom came running with a valium for him to take so he wouldn't feel upset. Once his grandmother, who was an emergency room nurse, overdosed and the toxicology report revealed she had taken the equivalent of 15-5mg Valium. To my surprise and disappointment, as it turned out, drug addiction was already a family secret and apparently, he had access to his grandmother's valiums for years.

Alcohol Hijacked Our Lives

When I first met his family, it looked perfect from the outside, but after I was in, all the family secrets of substance abuse was obvious. Still, it didn't dawn on me of how badly his family history of alcohol and drug abuse was going to affect our marriage, my life and my daughter's future until his drinking progressed into a dangerous habit. Unfortunately, the bigger family secret was that he was conditioned to substance abuse since childhood and if there is a gene that makes a person more prone to addiction he most likely inherited it. Additionally, the family had a deep belief that taking valium and other psychotropic drugs are acceptable to prevent feeling any stress or negative emotions, as long as it was a prescription medication, the problem was, he was also drinking heavily with the meds. In our early 20's our lives came crashing down as soon as he began mixing alcohol with nerve pain medication. He began having violent alcoholic blackouts at age 23 while I was 7 months pregnant, he came home at 2 a.m. drunk and I tried to speak to him about not drinking for the baby's sake and expressed that we needed to be more responsible now that we were going to be parents, he was drunk and feeling pressure from work, and now me. He snapped in an alcoholic blackout, he grabbed me and threw me across the bedroom, screaming don't pressure me I get enough pressure at work! Luckily, I landed on the side of the bed, otherwise he could have caused me to have a miscarriage. Soon after, he passed out. While I stayed awake trying to figure out what to do, I had always been taught if a man ever lays a hand on you, call the police and leave. I was 7 months pregnant and scared. I decided I was not going to confront him again about his drinking, while I was pregnant. I decided since I had some scholarship money I was going back to college and was going to finish my college education and go back to work so he wouldn't feel so stressed and so I could support my baby. While he was passed out from drinking, I had come to the clear understanding the he was not the man I thought I could depend on to support a family and live happily ever after with. The next day, he didn't even remember assaulting me and he wanted to take me down to the lake for a picnic like nothing ever happened. I loved him with all my heart but he had just had his first alcoholic blackout and I was frightened. Also, during that time, we lived on the outskirts of Memphis and within a couple of weeks I found out I had a stalker, a neighbors nephew had been stalking me and broke into our house while I was 5 months pregnant, the police were called and the man was arrested. I took the opportunity to move back home to prepare for the birth of our child in a more safe environment. We bought a place next door to his grandmother, the nurse, so she would be close by to help her and so she could help us with the baby. While apart, we made an agreement that he would control his drinking and only drink outside the home.

Stress Induced Relapse

During my seventh month of pregnancy, my grandmother died. My dad's mom was the closest one to my father that I had left and it was devastating to me to lose her before she could see my baby, her great granddaughter. Just after her funeral, we received a blessing. My husband's job transfer finally came through and we moved into a new home together living a block from his grandparents. We wanted to be close to so we could help them and they could spend time with our new baby. We set up the nursery together for our soon to come baby. He began going to lamaze classes with me we were excited and things seemed to be going smooth. The day came that I went into labor during a tornado warning. He drove me to the hospital with multiple tornados touching down all around us. It was a total drama. The tornado was blowing trees down blocking our path to the hospital. He had to stop and move trees off the road to clear the path to the hospital a couple of times. There were power lines down on the road and he had to drive over them in route to the hospital. I was in extreme labor pain and we were both in fear of the tornados sucking us up and away in the storm. At one point we saw a tractor trailer rolling over like a tumbleweed. Luckily we were in an aerodynamic sports car, white chickens were hitting the windshield that had blown out of the semi that was blown away, I thought the white chickens were a sign of the holy spirit. I was in labor, on my hands and knees praying in the seat of a sports car, in excruciating fear and pain and afraid we wouldn't make it to the hospital before giving birth. Everyone else was in their storm shelters, we were out in the storm trying to get to the hospital to have our baby. I insisted we go to the hospital and it's a good thing we did, from all the stress of tornados and the journey to the hospital, our baby was born at 2:00 a.m. a meconium baby, 5 on the apgar scale and luckily there was a neo-natal intensive care unit on site to save her life. His nerves were shook and he ended up not going in the delivery room with me and directly after her birth, he disappeared until a couple days later when he came to pick us up at the hospital.

2nd Relapse Rage

The storms had past and it was a bright sunny spring day, new life was springing up all around us and everything seemed wonderful for the 3 weeks as I was healing after the birth of our daughter. He was coming home every night and trying to live a normal life. I was utterly filled the with the joy of being a new mother of a beautiful happy baby girl, I was breast-feeding and getting to know my baby, while he was working everyday and out drinking every night. He was keeping the promise of doing it outside of our home but then 3 weeks after birth, he came home drunk, he had a bad day at work and was angry at the world and when I tried to calm him, he blacked out in a drunken rage and drug me around the house on the carpet until I had carpet burns and I was so weak from having the baby, in self-defense, I grabbed the only weapon I could reach and hit him in the head with a glass to get him off of me, then I grabbed our baby and fled to my mother's house. In route, I called my brother and I informed him what happened and he did a well check on him. As usual, the next day he did not remember any of what happened but he had a sore noggin and a hangover.

Our Family Intervention

I was very hurt emotionally, heartbroken and flat out tired of the domestic abuse during his alcohol blackouts. I was so afraid and disappointed. I refused to raise my child in that unstable environment so I left him and intended on divorcing him at that point. I stayed with my mother three weeks until I healed from my delivery and started to file the divorce papers, surprisingly he agreed to quit drinking and assured me love could keep our family together. My family was involved at that point, and insisted our safety was in jeopardy and that I needed to start thinking of mine and my daughters safety and make arrangements to secure our safety. I was only 19, had a small infant under a year old and I was in the process of filing papers for divorce but then he agreed to quit drinking, completely. I agreed to come back for the sake of trying to save our marriage. At the time, I was thinking that it was just bad behavior and that he would snap back into being my kind high school sweetheart. It wasn't just him being mean or bad behavior, it was some mental illness taking over his mind, addiction and alcoholism taking over his body and it was something bigger than what he was capable of controlling on his own, it was controlling him. It was a tolerable relationship, when he was sober and for short periods of time, then he would always relapse. He went through multiple relapses, each one progressively worse than the last and I was caught in a never ending hell.

Signs of Codependency

- Putting someone else first before yourself, usually someone who is abusive or neglectful in some way, such as an alcoholic or an addict.
- Staying in an abusive or neglectful relationship where your needs are not met or your safety is in jeopardy
- Having difficulty making decisions in a controlling relationship
- Having difficulty identifying and expressing your feelings
- Being bullied- having difficulty communicating in a relationship
- Valuing the approval of others more than valuing yourself
- Lacking trust in yourself and having poor self-esteem
- Allowing someone to abuse you fear of leaving the person
- The Stockholm syndrome / trauma bonding or terror bonding

Relapse Tragedy

There is a story behind every alcohol tragedy and when an alcoholic relapses the drinker is a tragedy waiting to happen. Our families were both involved in helping me with watching our daughter while I was in college and working part time. After a few weeks he appeared to be doing well with abstaining from drinking so we arranged for him to watch our daughter a couple of hours. One night, while I was in class, he was suppose to pick up our 3 ½ year old daughter from his mother's house, he had been off work and he showed up late and drunk an hour before my class was over. He had relapsed and I was so disappointed. He came to pick up our daughter from his mother's house but he was drinking again and drunk driving. His mom called me and I left class early, she asked me to hurry up and informed me that he is drunk, irrational and is insisting on and taking our daughter! I drove over there as fast as possibly could, but it was too late. By the time I got to the curve before his mother's house I saw the flashing red lights of the rescue squad, ambulance and police, as I got closer, i saw the whole area taped off, like a crime scene or a death scene and then my heart sank as I looked closer and saw his truck crashed head on into a large pine tree, I began crying and praying in fear, the pickup was demolished, totaled, the front end was crumpled up like a tin can and smoking, the tree was in the dash and the windshield was shattered, I was trembling with grief and dread as I got out of my car and ran up to the truck, in fear of finding my beautiful blonde baby girl amongst the wreckage and for a moment I realized something was terribly wrong, there were officers combing the wooded area around the wreck and I couldn't see my husband the truck was empty. I went up to the police and rescue workers swarming the scene and asked, "Where are the passengers? Are they alive"? The first responders said, we don't know, the passengers are missing, they could not find the passengers!

He fled the scene, leaving me to imagine the worst, in horror, I had no idea, where he or my baby daughter was, he vanished from the scene of the wreck I raced to my mother-n-laws house 1000 yards down the street in the worst fear and emotional pain you can imagine. For the first time, I hated him, I feared he had picked her up and that my baby girl was being rushed to the hospital or had been killed. When I arrived at my mother-n-law house she opened the door holding my daughter and much to my relief handed my baby to me safe and sound, she was ok. I felt so relieved. That night my mother-in-law did the best thing she ever did in her life, she refused to allow her son take our daughter in his drunken condition and therefore, she saved my daughter's life, that night we escaped death. She said, he came to pick her up but because he was drunk she refused to let him pick our daughter up and they even struggled and fought over taking his keys but he got away and drove off mad without our daughter and after he scratched out of the driveway and sped away as drove around the curve screeching wheels, she heard the loud boom of his truck hitting the pine tree and the glass and metal crashing, ironically, it happened in front of one of his father's best friends house.

Hide Keys Stop DUI Deaths

Apparently, his dad or a friend quickly arrived and pulled him out of the wreckage and drove him back to his mom's to hide in the basement to keep the police from arresting him on a DUI. When I saw him, he was hardly recognizable and it was the worst injuries I had ever seen on a living human being. He was drunk, hiding, refusing to speak to the police and refusing to go to the hospital, he was scalped from the windshield and had hematoma and multiple other injuries from the automobile accident. I was only 21 yrs young and his family told me, they had to work out a plan, they told me to go back to the wreck and tell the police it was my vehicle and that I was driving and lost control and hit the tree. I did and the police officer said, mam, I don't believe you, you have no injuries and if you were driving, where did you hide the body of the other passenger with brown hair scalped off in the glass of the windshield? After I claimed fault in the accident, the investigative officer walked me under the yellow crime scene tape, to our vehicle and shone the flashlight inside at the drivers side windshield, it looked like someones black haired toupe was stuck in the driver's side windshield glass.

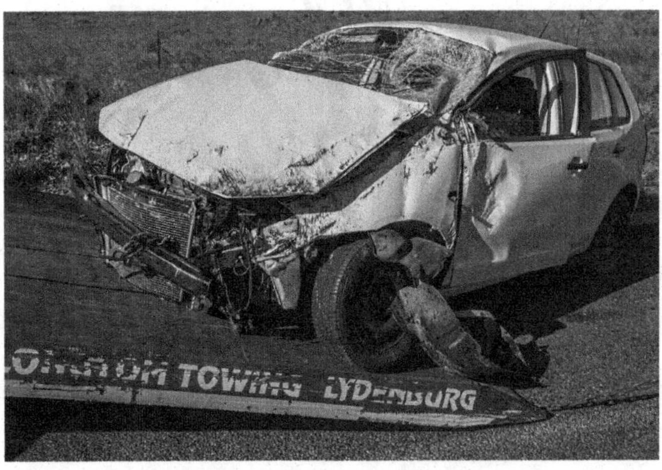

The truck was totaled. Had our daughter been with him she would not have survived the crash. I was just happy that she was alive and I was in shock from what almost happened to her. I was in shock and emotionally numb with fear and disappointment and just going through the motions like a brainwashed hostage.

The officer said, I see this vehicle is registered in your and your husbands names I am going to give you one chance to tell me the truth; where is the driver that wrecked this vehicle and are they alive?!? I clammed up, I told him I don't know and I couldn't think and that I thought maybe I was in shock. The officer then said, mam, I need an answer or I'm going to have to take you in for questioning and mam, before you answer, know this, falsifying a police report is an arrestable offence. I started crying and told them I don't know but likely it was my husband and that they needed to contact my father-n-law the deputy sheriff to find out where he was and then I gave the officer all of my contact information and our address along with my father-in-laws phone number and I asked him to please let me go check the hospitals and since my father-in-law was well known, they allowed me to go. I am sure they allowed me to go because his dad was a deputy sheriff, at the time, they were assuming maybe he picked up his son and took him to the hospital. Sure enough within minutes showed the police investigators showed up at my in-laws house searching for the missing injured driver. (unknowing the injured drunk-driver was hiding in the basement half-dead). The nightmare turned into a massive cover-up. My mother-in-law quickly convinced the police that his father, the deputy sheriff, had rushed him to a bigger hospital instead of the small local hospital and that they would come to the station for questioning as soon as he was checked out at the hospital and the police left. However, they did not take him to the hospital, they would not let me take him to the hospital and they had his grandmother, the ER nurse to check him and he did not go to the hospital, until the next day after the alcohol had worked its way through his system. You would think a drunk driver would quit after a wreck.

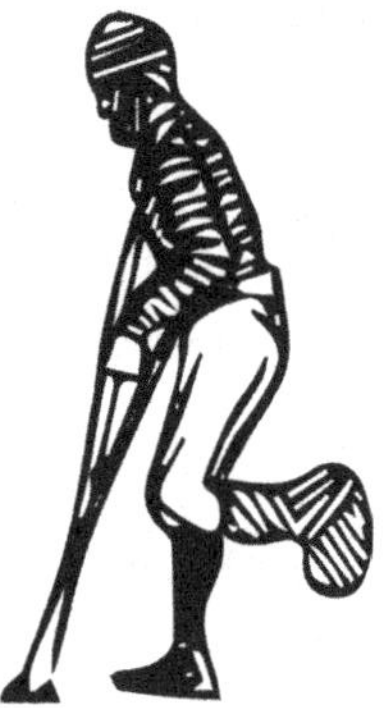

I Don't Have A Drinking Problem A Tree Jumped In Front Of My Truck!

The whole family had staged and participated in an elaborate cover up, which enabled him to get away with a serious drunk driving accident. I expressed, desire to commit him to rehab and expressed my worry that he could die from the large hematoma, skull fracture and infection. I expressed my disapproval and fear. I refused to take part in falsifying a police report. I pushed hard to sign him into rehab and they all cornered me like a pack of wolves. The majority ruled instead of an intervention, it was 3 against 1, an enablers cover-up meeting. They were completely enmeshed and it was negatively affecting our marriage.

Enmeshment:

A psychological term that describes a blurring of healthy boundaries between people, typically family members, when one person makes another person's problems, their own. Enmeshment often contributes to dysfunction in families and may lead to a lack of individuation, autonomy and independence that is unhealthy and can become pathological.

Emotional Incest

When a parent excessively exerts control over their child's mind rather than their body as is seen in physical incest. Healthy mental or emotional boundaries are crossed without physical sexual abuse. A parent uses a child as a surrogate spouse when that spouse is emotionally unavailable those emotions are flooded on the child which is emotional incest. Additionally, when a child is not allowed to resist being emotionally dumped on by the parent and not allowed to feel or express their own negative emotions. A parent may drug or medicate the child to suppress their emotional outburst. If a parent engages with administering or sharing a mood or mind altering medication, to control their underaged child or other family member to keep them under their control.

Family Enablers Blame Outsiders

Parents rarely blame their children for their own mistakes. A family may find it hard to point out its members individual flaws it's easier to blame the new member than to face the truth. I became their scapegoat. An alcoholic will divert attention off of themselves by bringing up the faults of other family members. Those in denial will say their drinking is not the problem, the family member that try to help the drinker quit, becomes the "nag" who is stressing the poor Alcoholic, the drinker will say its their fault that they drink to put up with the stress of being nagged. My in-laws told me that from now own, he would stay at home to do his drinking so he didn't get out and into anymore trouble drinking and driving or risk going to jail, rehab or lose his license, job or disgrace the family. Suddenly, they put the blame on me, and that I would have to start keeping my mouth shut and allow him to drink in the home they said, the wreck happened because I was in college and not at home, they were in denial and tried to make me out to be the bad guy, which was ridiculous. The wreck happened because he was drunk driving. That is typical for the alcoholic and their enablers to deny they have a problem and blame others for troubles that arise from their drinking problem. Their making enabling decisions in total disregard for me and my daughters needs and safety after I refused to enable this behavior revealed how immeshed they were and it was damaging to our marriage. I was forced into the position of an enabler with them silently keeping up appearances for a while, longer.

Silence Is A Virtue, Of An Enabler

Sobering Alcohol Related Child Deaths

According to the CDC, every day, 29 people in the United States die in motor vehicle crashes that involve an alcohol-impaired driver. The annual cost of alcohol-related crashes totals more than $44 billion. In 2016, 10,497 people died in alcohol-impaired driving crashes, accounting for 28% of all traffic-related deaths in the United States.

- There is one alcohol related auto death every 50 minutes.
- Of the 1,233 traffic deaths among children ages 0 to 14 years in 2016, 214 children died by the hands of an alcohol-impaired driver.
- There are 111 million self-reported episodes of alcohol-impaired driving incidents among U.S. adults each year.
- In 2016, more than 1 million drivers were arrested for driving under the influence of alcohol or narcotics.
- Drugs other than alcohol (legal and illegal) are involved in about 16% of motor vehicle crashes (the majority of crashes are alcohol related)

Fear In The Dysfunctional Family Of An Alcoholic

Within 3.5 years, of being married. I had been living in a constant state of fear and I finally gave up my hopes of being a happy, healthy family with him. I felt he had broken all of his promises, he was drinking and smoking in the house in front of our toddler and though I had her going to a church day care and pre-school, it was still a regular occurance of some dramatic crisis with his alcohol abuse and us having daily arguments over his drinking and our failing marriage. He was selfish and constantly worrying his parents and fighting with his dad. He tortured us with fear and worry. His mother and I were constantly having to hide his keys and fighting with him over not allowing him to drink in the home nor drunk drive. It was totally dysfunctional family situation with sometimes him disappearing on a binge for a few days at a time, leaving me afraid and worrying that he was wrecked or was dead somewhere or that he would come home in an abusive drunken state. Once while he was drunk, I came home to find him drunk holding a rifle to his own head, he had it propped between his feet and the barrel under his chin. I managed to talk him out of killing himself. Once, he held a gun to my head and when he sat it down, I picked it up and ran him out of the house with it then later the family confiscated his guns and hid them from him. Each time he was in an alcoholic blackout, he couldn't remember any of it the next day. He was a ticking time bomb. I tried several times, to convince just one family member to have the courage to co-sign with me to put him into rehab against his wishes and as each day passed he was in a constant state of agitation no one wanted to deal with him. Life was pure hell, torture and misery. It was killing his family to watch helplessly as he destroyed himself because we loved him, and yet none of us could trust him because he was also dangerous when he was under the influence of alcohol. No one in his family would help me commit him, they thought he would grow out of it before it got too serious. I watched alcohol completely transform the man who was my first boyfriend and high-school sweetheart into a grumpy, angry irrational drunk. Although, he was once a kind and loving husband he turned into a violent alcoholic who was destroying himself and his whole.

Alcohol Turns Some Drinkers Into Dr. Jekyll and Mr. Hyde

It was like dealing with two different personalities when my husband drank. We grew apart and he became an out of control stranger that I was afraid of what he was capable of doing under the influence. I came to the realization that it was not going to get any better. He was in a destructive vicious cycle of alcohol addiction. He was like a mouse caught in a trap repeating the same drinking behaviors in a never ending cycle over and over again.

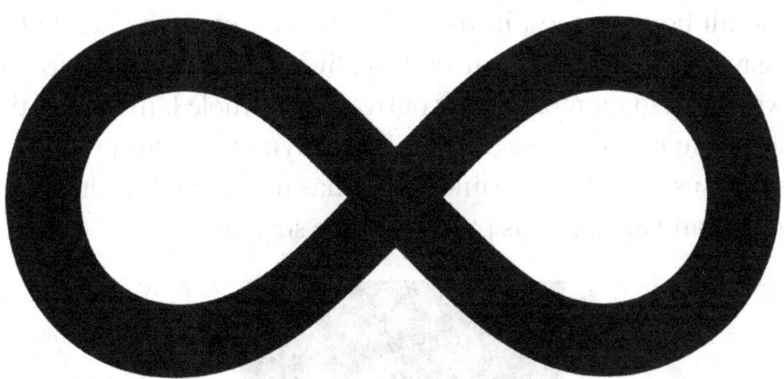

I became starkly aware that our lives were in a trap that was out of control and we were going nowhere in life because his only motivation was to have a drink. I had already almost lost my life and my daughter's life due to his violent drunk blackout episodes and irresponsible drunk-driving accident. I was in survival mode 99% of the time, at that point. It is a mother's natural instinct to protect her children. A sobering, thought was haunting me, every second; If my child had been in the car with her dad as she was suppose to be that night, she would have died. I became angry toward him for taking these risks and endangering our lives and I was growing bitter from his lack of responsible parenting. His actions had become totally unacceptable to me. Only a few years prior he almost caused me to have a miscarriage. Prior to experiencing these traumas, I had lost my own father in a tragic automobile crash, although no alcohol was involved with dad's accident, he had a blowout tire and hit a cement culvert on his way home from work and due to massive injuries, he bled to death before he could make it to the hospital. 10 years after my dad died in a car crash, I found myself worrying over my Alcoholic husband and wondering if he was going to die the same way that dad did. Every night he made it home, I was surprised.

Hope Dies Last

Even though we all survived his drunken rages and near death car crashes, our hearts were broken and the emotional wounds were mortal. There was no room left for denial. I was exhausted mentally, physically and emotionally from trying to love a man who could not and would not love himself, me or our daughter. It was like the good spirited person was gone and we were left with his ghost. He was only a shadow of the man, he used to be. It was a miracle he survived the wreck. His physical wounds and the scars on his face were healing but we all had permanent emotional scars from the trauma he was putting us thru and something died inside me that night, too, my hope died. My mom always told me, that once you've lost hope, you have nothing left. She was right, all hope was gone and there was nothing left to give me strength to carry on. Alcohol was a body snatcher and it grabbed him away from us and had his life in its full grip. All hope for things to get better, was gone. I lost all my trust in my husband to be a good father to our daughter and make wise decisions and all hope was lost in his ability to lead us as the head of our family. All hope was lost. I gave up trying to convince unwilling family members to co-sign him into rehab. Alcohol was like a giant monster in control of the whole family, and the family secret was out in the open. He refused to even try to quit anymore at this point and he was going to continue to torture us all with his drinking dramas no matter how it made any of us feel. He was like a puppet and alcohol was pulling all the strings.

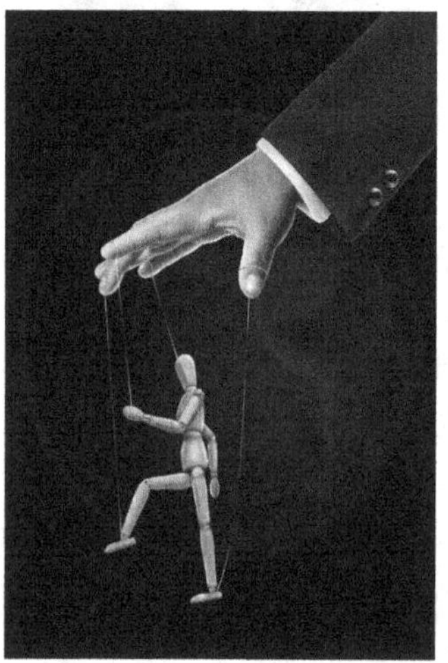

I was becoming emotionally numb and had to make a choice to quit being in the co-dependant relationship or stay and live a life spiralling out of control in hell on earth with him and always living in terror knowing that staying meant we would always be at risk of him creating a catastrophe or causing harm to us all. The family had been on an emotional rollercoaster with him for 3 years. He was an alcoholic and it was too late to turn back because at this point he refused to even try to quit, he loved drinking more than he loved us and even more after he almost died in the car wreck. A part of me died inside and though love is blind, my eyes were opened by his actions and I lost my empathy for him from the misery he put me through. I became emotionally numb to him after years of tears, disappointment and pain. I didn't feel loved or valued. His parents chose to be their son's enablers and they covered for him, always bailing him out and looking the other way. I asked his mom why, she wouldn't help me sign him into rehab so he could get help and so he could get clean and sober. She said, he was her only child and she was afraid her parents would find out and cut him out of the will for bad behavior. She also was afraid he would hate her for committing him, plus, she thought he would grow out of it, soon. He manipulated us into a triangle of enabling with his mother, it became a two against one game that I started refusing to play. He was 25, I was 22 I knew he wasn't going to just grow out of it.

Becoming An Alcoholics Enabler

- Includes ignoring or looking the other way
- Pretending and overlooking the alcohol problem
- Avoidance- avoiding "the talk" or an intervention
- Bailing the alcoholic out, repeatedly
- Taking the blame for the addicts drunken mistakes
- Protecting the Alcoholic when it puts yourself at legal risk
- Giving the addict another chance, too many times
- Ignoring the alcoholics problem and resistance to rehab
- Accepting constant irrational excuses and diverted blame
- Always being the one to clean up the alcoholic's mess
- Constantly, trying to fix the alcoholic's problems
- Continually coming to the alcoholic's rescue
- Never being supported always being used by the alcoholic
- Allowing the alcoholic to mow down your boundaries
- Allowing the alcoholic to abuse you and your relationship

His grandparents were wealthy from owning part of the Boston coal mines. It was a continual priority to hide their grandson's alcoholism. There were other unhealthy behaviors in the family, the grandparents were not substance abusers at all but they were staunchly religious and would put great pressures and high expectations on the family, basically keeping the family in financial servitude and always dangling the inheritance carrot to manipulate and control the family and they were always threatening to cut someone out of the will for not complying to their demands.

Manipulation is Always An Ongoing Mind Game In The Codependent Families Dynamic

Emotional Rollercoaster & Exhaustion

After 3.5 years, I was emotionally exhausted. Having an alcoholic partner is exhausting because they are unpredictable. If they are a binge drinker, they disappear often without explanation. It is exhausting because you can never sleep sound when they are missing. There is much suspense, presumably they're out drinking but they could be in jail or dead. They never come home on time and sometimes they don't come home at all. You constantly worry about where they are and if they are safe or if they are in trouble. When you hear an ambulance siren, you wonder if it is for them. When they don't show up you wonder if they are dead. When you hear a police siren, you wonder if they are being taken in on a DUI. They put you through so much pain, they spoil every special occasion by getting drunk and causing a scene that turns every holiday into an unhappy experience overshadowed by some disappointing drunken drama. Sometimes when they miss their own birthday party you may even wish they were dead so you no longer have to live in constant misery and worry. They put you through hell. Sometimes, you are surprised and delighted to see they have actually made it home alive. Life with an alcoholic is a constant emotional rollercoaster ride.

Alcohol had our lives on an out of control emotional rollercoaster, too. I would say my ex was drinking at least 55 % of the time we were together, from the middle of my pregnancy till the end of our relationship. After, I left, he made his mother into his enabler and over the years he fell deeper down into a bottomless pit of alcoholism, driving a wedge between every other family member. His dad and mom divorced. His parents would remarry and those marriages would end over their children interfering and because his step parents didn't agree with his parents codependent enabling and it caused disputes over money wasted to bail him out. It was a continual never ending recurring bail out. It was painful for us watching him ruin his life with alcohol from afar and he eventually ended up in trouble with the law and the judge forced him into rehab. Just like so many others, thc minute he was out of rehab, he was back drinking. 12- Step programs are great for some but never worked for him, he would get out, be around the same environment and relapse into alcoholism time and time again.

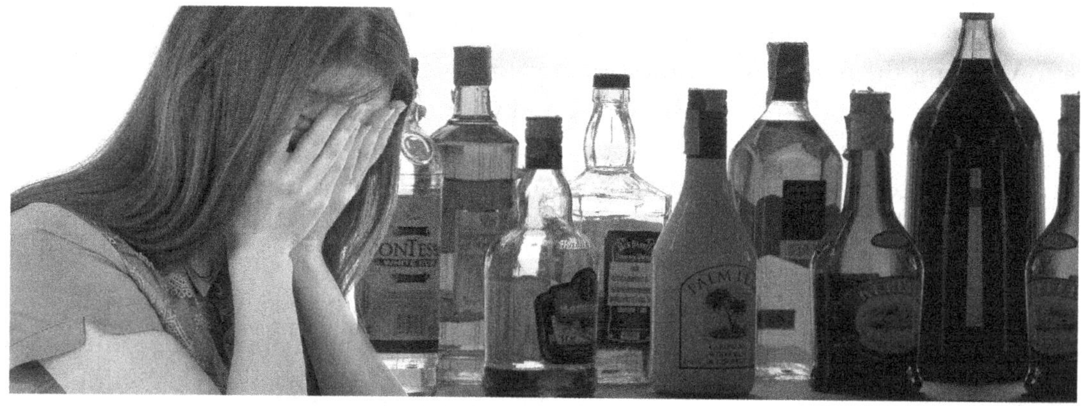

It is hard to share this, I want to give you an honest picture of the desperation of alcoholism and how it grips its victims and traps families in a cycle of grief.

Each Alcoholic Is One Of God's Children, & Deserving Of Help And A Second Chance In Life.

It's difficult to tell our story and keep it in a way that is respectful to him, his mother and daughter. His mom was very supportive to him, she was a kind, loving, giving and unwaveringly supportive mom. His daughter was kind, beautiful and sweet to him and neither one of us deserved to be put through the hell he put us all through with his drinking. Alcohol related problems plagued his whole adult life, drinking created one disaster after another throughout his entire adult life. Though he tried to quit, it seemed he never could. Living with an alcoholic loved one is a constant misery. He put us all through a living hell. His mother was afraid he would hate her for having him committed for treatment, instead they chose to wait hoping he would "grow out of it" on his own without the embarrassment of having to send their only son to rehab. Not signing a child into rehab as early as possible is the biggest mistake a parent can make. For some, it may not work, but it is always worth a try if you loved one is out of control with their drinking, and if they become a danger to their self or others.

Addiction & Alcoholism Is Not Something You Just Grow Out Of

Loved ones may enable the addict because they feel responsible for causing the substance use disorder. When a loved one has a substance use disorder, it is natural for families to want to fix the problem. While their intentions are seemingly good, family members who don't know the difference between helping and enabling may end up contributing to the addiction.

Enabling Behaviors From Family

However, there are several steps families can take to stop enabling and start helping. They often blame themselves for the addiction and try to make up for it by sacrificing time, money and energy. Family members make these sacrifices to reduce their loved one's pain and suffering, but they often don't realize they're engaging in enabling behaviors procrastinates recovery. Enabling behaviors come in many forms. For example, continually paying bail for the alcohol abuser, driving the alcohol abuser around after they've lost their license, taking the blame for fender benders on insurance claims and when enabling behaviors are enmeshed with codependency and other mental illness, the enabler will go over the line to participate in the addicts schemes to get money for booze or drugs, such as driving a getaway car or by providing a false alibi to help the addict cover up their crimes. By recognizing and ceasing these unhealthy codependent behaviors, families can gain back healthy boundaries, integrity and focus on getting their loved one into proper treatment program before the damage becomes irreparable.

Acknowledgement

One or more aquaintencences or family members of the drinker, acknowledge that the drinker may have a problem. Acknowledgement usually only happens after some problems related to alcohol arises in the life of the drinker

Denial

Denial is one of the primary behaviors that families adopt when they learn that their loved one is addicted to drugs or alcohol. They refuse to accept the reality that their family member has a substance use problem. They convince themselves that treatment isn't necessary and the addict will know how to control their drug or alcohol use or think they will grow out of it.

Justification

Justification and denial work hand in hand. Families often reject the problem, making up reasons to justify their loved one's addiction, and make up excuses for their child. For example, a family member may feel that it is fine for a loved one to use alcohol or drugs to cope after a break-up or a stressful day at work. Parents may also believe the substance use is only temporary and will stop after a change in lifestyle such as college graduation.

Allowing Substance Use

Family members may think that they are controlling the situation if they allow their loved one to drink or use drugs at home. They may even consume alcohol with the addict to manage their intake level and to make sure they gravitate toward home when using instead of more dangerous locations. It is better that home be the place to set an example for your children by having an alcohol free zone in the home.

Suppressing Feelings

Not talking about the problem, not expressing your concerns about addiction to a person you love gives them a reason to keep using. In some cases, substance users dismiss their families' fears by reassuring them that they will not consume drugs or alcohol.

When an addict dismisses these fears and concerns, it may encourage family members to keep their feelings to themselves.

Avoiding the Drinking Problem

By being passive or ignoring the problem and not confronting the substance user, family members may feel that they are keeping the peace in their home. Instead of getting their loved one proper treatment, the family focuses on keeping up appearances to look normal.

Protecting the Family's Image

The stigma of Alcoholism as substance use is ever present. People may be ashamed of their substance-using family members, leading them to portray the person in a falsely positive light to friends, co-workers and acquaintances.

Minimizing the Drinking Situation

People surrounding the addict may lighten the issue by convincing themselves that the substance user could be in worse situations. They treat the addiction as a phase that will improve on its own with time and patience.

Playing the Blame Game

Adopting negative attitudes toward substance users only pushes those struggling with addiction away. Blaming or punishing individuals for their substance use alienates them from their family, which may result in destructive behaviors.

Enabling or Assuming The Drinker's Responsibilities

Family members may be inclined to take over the regular tasks and responsibilities of the addict in an effort to prevent their lives from falling apart. Instead, assuming responsibilities and providing money to the substance user removes accountability and allows them to fully indulge in their addiction.

Confronting and Controlling Behaviors

Exerting control on a substance user may worsen their addiction. Constantly treating the addict as an inferior or placing numerous restrictions on their lifestyle may drive them further from the family unit and closer to their substance-using peers.

My Short Life With An Abusive Alcoholic

Our life was a textbook case of all of the previously mentioned unhealthy family enabling dynamics of alcoholism and codependency. Life was getting worse by the day until it became an unlivable environment to raise a child in. I realized that we were dealing with a dual diagnosis, in addition to alcoholism, some type of mental illness was presenting. After a few more of his destructive tantrums and often violent alcoholic blackouts. I realized our lives were in danger and he was out of self-control and no matter how many times he said he would quit. I was in fear of our lives, and each blackout was worse and worse than the last one. He once stabbed me in the hand. Another time, he put a cigarette on on my lips, because I didn't allow smoking in the house around the baby. Another time, he drug me around in the house like a rag-doll, another time he banged my head into the concrete floor of the garage until I had black eyes and a concussion the next day. Another time he burned my clothes he said I looked to good in them. The harder I worked to pull his end of the load and the more successful I became the worse his jealousy, mental illness and alcoholism became. It was devastating and heartbreaking, and the sad thing is, he always claimed he did not remember any of his abuse because every time he did those hurtful things, he was in a total alcoholic blackout. I was in love with him, I thought we would be together forever, we had a small child, we had plans to build our dream home by the creek on our land. I never wanted to end up divorced. It was a last option and I didn't quit on us, easily.

Addiction Is More Dangerous For The Family Members Than The Addict, Themself

At that point, It wasn't even about that we had different value systems, he was a dangerously violent alcoholic. As a mother, I refused to raise my child in that environment or continue to allow an alcoholic to be the primary male role model for my daughter. He was not helping, he was hurting. He tried to quit, but each time it would be 3 days or 3 weeks and he was back on the bottle and progressively getting worse in every imaginable way. He was hooked and he just didn't have the inner strength to kick the habit on his own and wouldn't get professional help to quit. I could not connect with him anymore, none of his family could convince him to quit. I was miserable he started not coming home at night because I didn't want him drinking, or being mean and violent, in front of our daughter. His drinking was affecting his work, he had received a few warnings from his supervisors and I was trying so hard to fix everything to take the stress off him, I was dying inside, but somehow I was doing well at work, getting recognized for exceeding the company's expectations of me and making more money than he was and he had insecurities about it.

Holidays With An Alcoholic

The Holiday season is "binge season" for the typical Alcoholic. The last and final straw of my life being married to an alcoholic was on christmas eve, his mother had spent the night with us to help me prepare holiday desserts for our family christmas dinner the next day, and he stayed out drinking and did not come home until 2 am. We had went to bed around 11 pm and were fast asleep waiting on santa claus to come home for our daughters 3rd christmas. My mother-in-law had out of habit, locked the screen door but all hell broke out when "santa-clause" could not just slip in unnoticed after a night of drinking with the boys, he woke us all up screaming in a drunken stooper to let him in and he was very angry that he had been locked out. When I opened the door "santa clause" was in a rage and immediately blamed me, he began screaming and swearing at me chasing me around the island in our kitchen, he was obviously drunk and amped up on some kind of drugs, he took off his big black cowboy boot and threw it at me and it went straight through the sheetrock into the wall by the christmas tree, just inches from my head.

It 'Twas The Night Before Christmas & Santa Was A Naughty Drunk!

His mom came from our daughters bedroom into the kitchen and stepped in the middle in between us saying son, calm down because it was her who accidently locked the screen door before we all laid down for bed for the night, but, as she approached him, he grabbed his own mom and slung her across the room where she fell across the presents and into the living room coffee table and cracked her forearm which immediately swole up the size of a grapefruit. Just as his mom cried out in pain, as I ran over to help her up, my little 3 ½ year old daughter came out of her bedroom screaming daddy, I want you to stop being mean. Why are hurting my mommy and granny? Stop right now you are being scary! I picked her up and hugged her and said yes, daddy, Santa claus is coming and he can see you are not being nice! We all began to hug her and comfort her, it was the only thing that snapped him out of his alcoholic rage, at least she got him to laugh and then he past out after exhausting us all. His mom and I cleaned up the presents and I iced her arm. When daylight broke the next morning, his mom was at the ER getting x rays of her arm on christmas day and it was the worst christmas morning of our lives. His mom's arm was badly bruised, she had a hairline fractured radius bone and hematoma, by then it was swollen up the size of a softball. He was hungover and didn't remember a thing. So while the rest of us endured great emotional pain he enjoyed alcohol amnesia. It was a fatal blow to my love and all trust was shattered, forever. I knew if he could beat up his own mother, he was capable of killing me and our daughter. Little girls are a precious, a gift from god, a wife is also a blessing. He was such an alcoholic that he ruined the last thing we had left, our holiday family time.

Alcohol Ruined Our Dreams

On that christmas day, day we did not tell his dad or the rest of the family. Now, his mom and I were keeping secrets for the abusive alcoholic, technically we were enabling our abuser. His mom and I both were in so much pain and exhausted but our daughter seemed fine and was enjoying all of her new Christmas toys. The day after christmas, I had an intervention talk, with my father-in-law, the deputy sheriff, about his son had been assaulting me and his mom and that the baby had seen the assault and much to my surprise, instead of offering to help me sign his son into rehab, he said he thought it would be best for our safety at this point, for me to seperate and file for a divorce. Also, he said he would testify on my behalf for full custody. For the next 5 days, I talked to my boss at work and she helped me put in a job transfer within the company to a larger city 70 miles north. I found an apartment close to my sister, who had just moved back from Germany. Everyone knew my ex's alcohol abuse spiraled out of control and that our lives were potentially in danger and everyone, including his father helped me and our daughter escape to safety. He had become so out of control and violent and I was afraid of what he would do after I left. We all were afraid that he could snap and kill us all. He refused rehab and I refused to allow the violence be a part of our lives or home environment any longer. I secretly went to file for the divorce with an emergency protective order for full custody, he was unaware of my plan. On New Years Eve night, my daughter and I went to sleep in her room while her dad stayed up drinking, at 2.am. my 4 year old daughter woke me up shaking. I ask are you cold, she whispered no, daddy was holding a gun to your head and I assured her everything was going to be ok that we were going to have a happy new life soon and she would be around her cousins and get to play with them everyday. I woke up early on New year's day to discover his gun propped up against the wall by her bedroom door, I can only imagine what he almost did to us that night. I did not confront him about the incident, and when he left to go deer-hunting and my family was waiting down the street and rushed to help, me move out without notice. I will never forget, having to leave my home, as a young single mom, the disappointment is unimaginable and unless you have lived through a divorce, it's hard to explain. Usually, if you were going to break up with someone you would sit down like adults and talk it over and come to an agreement, eye-to eye and face to face, but not with a violent alcoholic. It was apparent there was more involved than alcohol and our arguments with him over his drinking, only pushed him closer to his addict friends outside the family. He was paranoid and having hallucinations and accusing me of all kinds of crazy fantasies. The last days of living with a violent alcoholic is like walking on eggshells in fear of setting off a landmine. Having to tip-toe in your own house and having to sneak out the door without setting off a booby-trap, this time it was forever.

Alcohol Triggers Dormant Mental Illness

My Silent Exodus

I left silently, as to avoid conflict, there was nothing to talk about anymore, and I realized I was not leaving the man I loved I was leaving the evil violent twin, the addict that had body-snached my sweetheart. I already learned talking didn't work and was a potential trigger. My job transfer was approved and I was done living in his hell. I was so hurt and filled with bitterness. I didn't understand what happened to his personality. I didn't understand mental illness or addiction. I was standing there in our empty house, there was a big red bow left over from one of my daughters christmas gifts and I stuffed into his empty 5th of vodka bottle, that he drank the night before on new years eve and I left a goodbye note beside the bottle stating he would have to quit for us to be a family again. I felt I had exhausted all the other options in my power so I made the "quit or die" decision. I chose to quit the relationship before he killed us in one of his drunken rages.

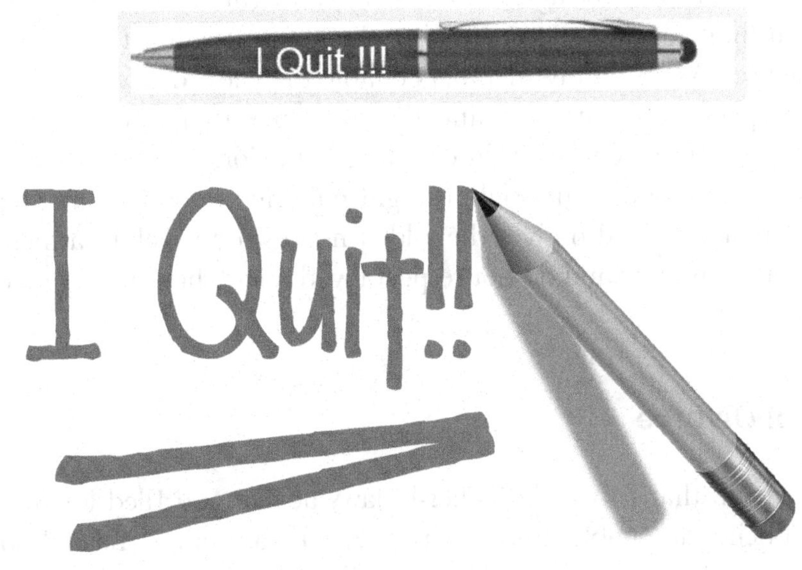

"I Quit Us Until You Quit Drinking"

That was the point, our marriage was mortally wounded. He killed my love for him. I realized our lives were never going to be normal. Because of alcohol, he was not the same person. I could not trust him to be the responsible leader of our family. I could not trust him in the care and safety of his own daughter. I had to turn to other people for love and support because he wasn't giving us any. I could not risk him having another alcoholic blackout and injuring our daughter like he hurt me and his own mother. At this point, he was more dangerous and violent than ever and he probably belonged in a rehab asylum. He had already gone too far and he was going to either kill us all or himself or both. I QUIT being an enabler to an alcoholic and my daughter and I both went through counseling to help us heal from all of the trauma. Everyone envisions their dream of what a perfect family life would be like. Mine was like the movie, "It's a Wonderful Life". Unfortunately, our lives were more like "A Nightmare Before Christmas" which, sadly, was our daughters favorite christmas movie after our nightmare christmas. I never told my daughter santa is coming on Christmas eve, ever again. It has been 30 years and we have had many wonderful holidays since to be grateful for, but for me, there is always the sting of the memory of the worst christmas of our lives when I was trapped in a relationship with an abusive alcoholic.

Enabling Alcoholism

Codependency is a behavioral condition in a relationship where one person enables another person's addiction, poor mental health, immaturity, irresponsibility or under-achievement. Enabling occurs when the friends and family of an alcoholic or substance abuser support the addiction through their actions, thoughts or behaviors. People who enable act as a cushion for addicts, preventing them from facing the consequences of their substance abuse. When family members enable their loved one's addiction, the co dependent loses respect for themselves, and the substance user loses respect for them, too. Ignoring the problem or engaging in enabling behaviors makes us lose self-respect because we know we're not doing the right thing. Enabling not only creates a permissive attitude toward drug use, but also gives the addict no desire to seek treatment. Enabled addicts lose faith in themselves and do not respect loved ones who make it easier for them to continue using drugs.

My Alcohol Divorce

I loved us so much, that I took my father-in-laws advice and filed for the divorce to break the cycle of being an enabler and codependent. I was young and did not have the best understanding of what alcoholism really is nor did I have the emotional skills to cope with the relationship. I felt that he loved drinking more than he loved his beautiful family that god had blessed him with. Me leaving only made him more out of control he began making death threats toward me. I had to go into hiding. I had to move to another region. He threatened my life, I will never forget those words. He said: "When I find you, I will kill you, I am going to slit your throat and pull your face off over your skull!" The grounds for our divorce was irreconcilable differences, due to his violent alcoholism, physical, verbal and emotional abuse. I was finally, free from my abuser. Still, for years he threatened me. And for years he blamed the divorce on me and my "driving him to drink" by leaving and involving outside health professionals, family and friends outside of our marriage to advise me on the healthiest way to deal with my and my daughters situation.

An Alcoholic in Denial Plays Blame Games

Many times the Alcoholic is in denial, and refuses responsibility for their actions. He had a double life, one with his drinking buddies and one with us. He refused to take any responsibility for how his behavior was affecting everyone around him, instead, he would say he didn't have a problem and insisted that everyone else, did. He blamed the whole family, his job, the dog and the cat and stress for driving him to drink. He denied any responsibility for his actions and insisted it wasn't his fault, it was ours, in his opinion. Our divorce occurred because of his abusive alcoholism. He refused to seek help or go to rehab to improve. He was working through some very angry emotional issues and was taking them out on me. We had a brick wall between us because he could not open up to me or anyone, emotionally. He was secretive he wouldn't confide in me as his spouse. I never understood why or what exactly was the cause of all of his hidden emotions and anger issues. Therefore, I could not help him so I had to help myself and my daughter. I felt like I did not know him anymore and could not relate to the person that alcohol had made him become and as long as he refused counseling, we could not come back or reconcile.

Guilt & Shame

Shame is just one challenge for the survivors of alcoholics. But it's nothing compared with the guilt. Sometimes, leaving a codependent relationship is enough to get the alcoholic to agree to rehab. Our leaving did not motivate him in the least to quit. It was like he was in love with another woman, only he wasn't, he was in love with a bottle, well not the bottle but the Alcohol in the bottle. Alcohol was his most important companion. My husband had an affair with alcohol and he left his family for "Alco-her", he was emotionally, physically, mentally in love with "Alco-her". I divorced my husband because he was having a long-term affair with Alco-her and he wouldn't stop. The shame of feeling like we were not worth it for him to quit alcohol to save us or that somehow he loved "Alco-her" more than he loved us. He didn't think that me and our daughter was as important as having a drink. The hurt, the shame and guilt is the most painful thing the alcoholic puts their family thru. The alcoholic spouse will try to make you think you are not good enough, or worthy enough of love and happiness, but that's just a lie they try to get you to believe so you stay with them and put up with their abuse. I tried so hard, I just could not say or do enough to convince him to quit drinking to save his family and our marriage. I was filled with despair, it was unbearably heartbreaking and painful. For those of us who have lost a spouse to Alcoholism the guilt is also painful, we are the ones who gave up, we left them and they were sick with a seemingly incurable disease. However, I feared if I didn't leave he was going to kill us all or I would accidentally kill him in self-defense during one of his violent blackouts. I couldn't put my child through that. I left, and tried not to talk badly about him, because my daughter. No one knows what goes on behind closed doors, and I had done a good job of hiding "his problem" to friends in the community. He turned in to this party going bad-guy divorcee, and since he was strikingly good looking (he looked kind of like Johnny Depp in those days) but he had anger issues and wanted to hurt me for leaving him, so he systematically tried to get close or date the other women in my circle, he even cornered my little sister in a bar and tried to kiss her and then went out with about 3 of my girlfriends, there was no shortage of women who would go out with him a few times before they figured it out he was a violent alcoholic and then they left him, too. He had a new relationship with another fitness trainer who looked strikingly similar to me, blonde, athletic and leggy. She called me one night hysterical and warned me that my life was in danger. She told me the night before that my ex had gotten drunk, was having an alcoholic blackout and shot a hole in the ceiling when she tried to leave, he chased her around the yard screaming at her and calling her by my name and telling her she had better get back there. She said, she had to hide in a drainage ditch to keep him from shooting her. I knew what his girlfriend told me was true and I knew it would have been happening to me had I stayed with him. I did everything I could to try to save him at some point a mother has to save herself and her child. There where numerous other incidences until he got into rehab, then he did better, he had a good relationship with a lady who had 3 kids and my daughter loved those times visiting her dad after his rehab and we knew there was hope for him in the future if we could get him into a rehab program that would better help him with lifelong sobriety. Unfortunately, he had a few relapses afterwards. I could write a movie about his life and it would be a very dramatic film. I don't feel shame or guilt anymore, that is how the disease destroys families and we have to get over the stigma of alcoholism so we can help each other understand and heal as a nation.

Our Family Is Not Alone

In addition to my own family tragedies, Addiction is 50% due to genetic predisposition and 50% due to poor coping skills. I have witnessed numerous instances of other people and their families also experiencing a myriad of emotions, loss and deaths of loved ones from alcohol use, abuse and alcohol related accidents. Numerous automobile fatalities, numerous over consumption issues. There is a story behind every alcohol tragedy and is is usually related to unmanaged or improperly managed emotional issues. It is not about the alcohol, it's about the self-medication with alcohol.

Signs Of Alcohol Abuse When Help Is Needed:

- Increased arguments at home with a spouse or significant other due to choices made under the influence or
- Disagreements over drinking and the negative impacts caused by alcohol abuse
- Difficulties at work that range from showing up late or calling in sick due to being unable to function at optimum levels

- Causing others emotional trauma related to alcohol abuse
- Impaired state of mental health
- Health problems related to mental health symptoms or alcohol abuse such as insomnia, poor eating habits, and chronic illnesses related to alcohol and inability to control drinking
- Mental health issues that impact others, including changes in personality or extreme/violent mood swings
- Any choices related to alcohol abuse such as drinking and driving
- Ongoing mental health symptoms such as suicidal behaviors or violent outbursts that put the person or others at risk.

Sometimes, rehab is the only viable option. Even though it may seem harsh and deliberately unhelpful, sometimes, a loved one has to be the one to kick the crutch right out from under the alcoholic. Alcohol is an emotional crutch. The codependent family will not take the crutch away from the alcoholic. Metaphorically, the crutch being the alcohol and kicking the crutch would be the equivalent of signing the alcoholic into rehab against their will for forced institutionalized treatment.

Involuntary Hold & Welfare Check

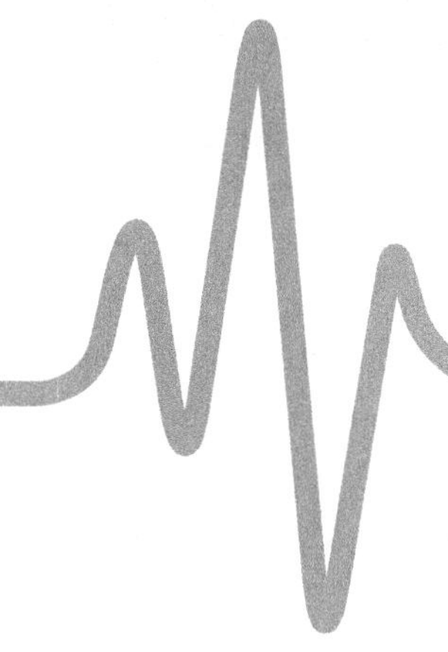

Chapter 8

Interventions

If you have a loved one who is having a mental health crisis and are clearly on a path of self-destruction with alcohol and they may also have unknown emotional disturbances or a psychiatric condition, you get them in for a psych evaluation, before it is too late. In some states it only takes one person to seek help for a family member. In other states, it requires two. If another family member will not help you sign them in to rehab, you may be able to file a 5150 for an adult or a 5585 for a teen psych evaluation. You could save your loved ones life by getting them help. Additionally, if you encounter homeless people, there are social services programs to help them, many times a 5150 is the best option to get homeless people off the streets into the proper mental health treatment program.

Alcohol Prevention Methods

There is no surefire way to prevent alcohol use. However, there are preventive measures that will likely reduce the consumption rate:

- Proper education that raises awareness about the actual risks of alcohol abuse. Education should be the first step in any harm prevention program and that education must begin early.
- While banning alcohol altogether is ideal, for some is an improbable scenario, creating curfews for alcohol serving and consumption that target the specific periods when alcohol-related crimes are the most prominent can have a positive impact.
- Creating free or very affordable and accessible public health rehabilitation system for those addicted to alcohol can help those with chemical dependency make a successful transition back into society, eliminating their need to depend on criminal activities to fund their alcoholism or addiction.

Healing My Own Codependency

I had to grow up at age 10, when my father died. I did not process the grief from the loss of my father though my childhood or teens. I brought the unhealed pain into my marriage. I lived in that nightmare of being married to an alcoholic for 3 ½ years. When my marriage was over I felt shattered. I felt totally let down by life and was emotionally wounded and disappointed that we did not have our "happily ever after." Also, I felt angry toward him for not loving us more than alcohol and for those last few weeks I don't believe he was completely sober a single day. I had so many unresolved issues. I could not stay in the marriage, the emotional roller coaster was killing me, I quit allowing him to force me into the position to play the role of the codependent enabler. I was hurt from not being appreciated and that he abused his power as a father and husband. I was not happy with my life. I felt that the relationship was changing me into an unhappy person. I did not want my daughter to become, fatherless, especially since my father had died in a car crash. I was angry that he was such a bad father and husband. I was angry at my dad for leaving me as a child and dying and not being there to protect me or meet my daughter and be in her life. I was angry at her father who was drinking and driving, though he never had a DUI at that point. I would not allow him to drive me anywhere. I did not trust him. I didn't want him risking others lives, either. I felt I was losing myself and my usually bubbly personality. My child was afraid. It was much worse but I will spare you the details, anyone married to an alcoholic can tell you pretty much the same story. It was a dangerous situation and it was inevitable that we divorce. He couldn't change his alcoholism without help and he refused help. I realized his relationship with alcohol was more important to him than his relationship with me. We were in misery. I could not be his enabler any longer. I could not save our family, I could not save him. I chose to save my daughter and myself. I chose the only option left, I walked out. When I told my mother-in-law, I was leaving her son, she said something that many loved ones of alcoholics say, "Don't leave I don't think I can handle him on my own. I can't handle his drinking on my own, either." Neither one of us could handle him and his mom thought he would straighten up for the sake of his daughter. Usually, a parents love is the strongest love, it is unconditional and he did love his daughter with all his heart unconditionally, but alcohol was in control over him above and beyond everything else. He was an alcoholic and I a codependent enabler who wasn't in the position to help him because I was angry and growing emotionally numb. The whole situation was killing me.

Enabling Is Not Love

As a mother, love is blind, we see no wrong in our children, we give them every benefit of the doubt after all they were our precious innocent babies, perfect in every way, from the outside. As mom's we pray for a healthy baby during pregnancy, when they are born with 10 fingers and toes and a fully functioning brain and body, there is no greater blessing in the world. As mom;s we nurture our children, teach them to be careful of dangers and how to be safe and avoid accidents. We teach them to avoid strangers, and to not get mixed up in the wrong crowd and to go for their dreams and try to build self confidence in them so one day they grow up and make a contribution to the world and hopefully, bless you with grandchildren, if that is what they want. I know it was hard for his mom, to admit her son had a problem. I didn't blame her. She didn't understand that they were enmeshed and she was his victim, too, as he had made her his enabler, since the wreck. In hindsight, it's easy to see thru his family history and understand the once hidden causes. So many people make the same mistake, mistaking enabling as love. Love is not helping to cover up the mess of a loved ones addiction, that is enabling. Bailing a love one out on a 1st time DUI, with the agreement they will quit and go to rehab is helpful but if you are bailing the same person out after their 2nd - 10th DUI it is not love, it is enabling. At some point we have to love someone enough to stop enabling them. Family counseling is imperative and sometimes tough love is necessary in dealing with an addict. Love is leaving an alcoholic to make room for them to learn to accept responsibility for their own actions. Love is to quit enabling the alcoholic's destructive behaviors so they take responsibility for their actions. Love is signing someone into rehab against their will, If they can't quit on their own so they can find out why they drink and hopefully have a better future. Love is knowing that your intervention is an important way of showing you care that they will have the chance to make it into rehab to change before they die. If they can't quit and they are violent or abusive then, pray for them daily, but remove yourself because they can hurt you or even kill you while in an alcoholic blackout or violent rage. If they dont quit drinking they will eventually meet their maker and it won't be under natural circumstances. Expect catastrophe. That is the life you will live with an addict and alcoholic. Its devestatenly heart breaking for everyone who loves them to watch them spiraling out of their own control.

Signs Of The Enabler

Being the codependent enabler is watching the person you love climb aboard a train that you know is going to wreck and you don't do anything to stop them. Enabling isn't love it is murder. All you will be left with is the wreckage and catastrophic aftermath and years of shame and guilt because you were not able to save them from themself.

The signs you may be a codependent enabler:

- You pick up booze for the alcoholic
- You call their work and lie that the alcoholic is sick so they don't get fired when in reality they are hung-over from the night before
- You are unhappy but you put the alcoholics needs before yours
- you sabotage your own methods of survival
- you put the other person first even if they are abusive to you
- your health or career suffers because of them
- You allow yourself to be abused
- You allow emotional or physical abuse of the alcoholics children
- You resort to extreme manipulation to keep the other person sober
- You are so caught up in the users game of wanting you to help them that you have no idea what your real feelings and needs are

- You are so over burdened with the alcoholics wants that you don't know what you want anymore
- You are depressed, exhibiting low self esteem/ self care/ self neglect
- Low self-esteem from not being valued
- Belittled by an alcoholic or abuser
- Suffer extreme feelings of guilt for the children
- Blame yourself for not being able to cure the alcoholic
- Feeling that if you were good enough, the alcoholic would quit
- Taking the blame for the alcoholics behavior
- You do not set healthy boundaries with other people
- Indulge in obsessive behaviour- think about your partner non-stop,
- Worrying and wondering what trouble they maybe getting into
- Constantly checking in on them, spying on them, you have lost trust
- You are taking on their responsibilities and bailing them out
- You feel you are being victimised, but if fact you are enabling them
- Believing you are powerless to change your situation
- You think things are being done 'to' you instead of tolerated by you

If you are the spouse of an abusive alcoholic, you may feel you have been forced into the role of being codependent. It's important for you to not only to help get counseling for the alcoholic, but also support for yourself and the children, too. Family counseling may help you make wise decisions, save your family or help to make the impending major life changes, such as divorce, as smooth of a transition as possible.

Who Is Affected By Alcohol?

The whole population has been involved or touched by alcohol on some level. Utilizing the information of public health organizations may help save yourself and your loved ones life and family. In most cities, there are state and local resources available to help you. Additionally, rehab facilities are a great source of information and in and out patient programs for alcohol recovery.

Living In Heavy Alcohol Use Communities

Environmental exposure to alcohol abuse increases your own risk of alcoholism. At 23 years old, I was going through a separation, divorce and child custody battle. I had been working in chiropractic healthcare as an xray technician and got a job in radiology in the ER at the local hospital. Sure enough, two of my first patients where alcohol related accidents, there was no running away from the heavy Alcohol use problem in our community. My first patient was a 16 year old, who had just got her license and a drunk driver hit her head on, the x ray revealed she had a broken neck and was paralyzed, another child's life shattered from alcohol. A few nights later, I am doing another emergency x ray on a man who had a gunshot wound to the abdomen, he was drinking with his buddy who accidentally shot him! I couldn't take the stress seeing the effects of alcohol ruining the lives of many of these emergency room patients. Working in the ER is extremely stressful, as you are dealing with tragedies on a constant continual basis. It made my problems seem like they weren't so bad in comparison. Internally, all the emotions were compounding. I wanted to get away from dealing with the problems of alcoholics, too. I learned I am too empathetic to work in ER, I felt their pain and I needed to be in a happier state of mind, so, I began researching into the field of wellness care. I began studying alternative healthcare and psychology. After doing my emotional work, I worked through many repressed emotions and as I got better, I decided to make a career out of helping others through wellness healthcare. I began working in chiropractic and went to college. I quit the job in the ER and began studying integrative medicine, functional medicine, behavioral medicine, naturopathy, psychology, mental health, alcoholism, addiction and codependency to try to understand why my family and all these other families were plagued with the negative crisis related to alcohol abuse. I realized that most people use alcohol as an escape mechanism from the pain and suffering of the human condition. I began to recognize this in my patients and encouraged them to take control of their lives, just as I had to adjust to our major life change to have a better life.

Church and Family Counseling

My daughter and I left the alcohol infested community, we got out alive and due to my ex's violent alcohol problem the judge awarded me full custody and he got weekend visitation every 2 weeks. We started a better life in a city 75 miles away. We joined a church and I was a sunday school teacher. We did some family counseling. Sadly, children have a more difficult time of escaping an alcoholic parent and her dad continued spiraling deeper into his alcoholism. The trauma we experienced caused separation anxiety. I worried about her and she worried about me when we were apart.

Forced Visitations With Parents & Alcohol Use

In many states, the courts force children of divorce to split time between parents and often children are traumatized by being shuffled between parents like a pawn in a chess game. Although I had full custody, the judge mandated she to go to visitations with her other parent. In those days, while the drinking was a factor, still children had to go visit their parents. Once when our daughter was 5 years old, during their weekend visitation, a family friend spotted my ex leaving a BBQ pool party drunk driving with our daughter standing up in the front seat. By the time I drove there, my mind was flooded with terror again over him risking the life of our daughter, while drunk driving. Upon arriving, I found he miraculously made it home but I had to step over a friend of his passed out on the floor to retrieve my daughter. Afterwards, I filed emergency protective orders and the child custody judge, agreed with me that environment was no place for a little girl. The judge would only allow her dad supervised visitation while his mother was present during all visits and from that point forward it was mandatory. He made the mistake of getting drunk again while she was on visitation and I called the police and had him arrested when he did not return her after a visitation. I was no longer his enabler after that. I no longer felt frightened for my daughters safety around him because afterwards the judge also ruled that his mom must be present during visitation and no alcohol use was allowed while she was with him on visitation or all visitation would be banished via court order.

Healing The Wounds

I loved my daughter more than anything in the world and I felt so badly for her to be mandated by the court to go to visitations and there was nothing I could do to stop court ordered visitation. It killed me that she may be exposed to her dad being drunk and driving her around. Many children are forced to go to visitations and there is no sober adult there to protect them. I spent most of my adult life always trying to make it up to her for the bad start we had in life, with him. I worked hard to make up for the unstable home life that we started out with. We lived in a rented condo for 2 years while I worked and made the money to buy land and built a home for me and my daughter, those were happier days, she chose the land to build our home when she was 6 years old and we built our new home and moved in when she was 7 years old. I raised her in that home until she was 18 and she had a more normal childhood with lots of happy times there. For me, it was a life of hard work, blood, sweat, tears and lots of love. Many of those years where spent making up for the trauma of earlier years. My main focus was providing a stable home environment for my daughter, working hard to give her a better life, going to church, teaching sunday school and keeping lots of family and friends around to help my daughter feel socially open, confident and stronger. My daughter made many friends at her new school and she had birthday parties with lots of kids games and pool parties, lots of sleep over's with dozens of other little girls and boys for her to play with. We focused on the positive experiences in life. I did the best I could to be a better mom and our families, church family, friends and neighbors were supportive of us, too, which helped create a much needed, safe environment for my daughter to grow up in.

At age 11, the judge ruled that my daughter would no longer be forced to go to supervised visitation with her dad and she could decide when she wanted to visit. That was a relief when visitation came on her own terms. I tried to keep her busy with her own personal growth. I enrolled her in a private school in the 6th grade though jr. high, where she had more one-on-one attention from her teachers, smaller class rooms, art classes along with basic education. It was a less stressful environment. Our neighbors kids were into swimming so we enrolled my daughter in lessons and soon after she began competing in swim team competitions, this helped build her self confidence and she flourished and in touch with her individual self interest. I was proud to see her develop her own interest and for a little girl, she worked hard on her swimming skills and became the champion at breast stroke in her class and division. She was a winner and won several competitions and even made it to state and regional competitions. She also, did plays and musicals at the church and schools, she took singing lessons, piano lessons, saxophone lessons and was in the choir. As a pre teen she took acting lessons and joined the river-bend players where she did peer-pressure prevention plays at local schools to help fellow teens to raise behavioral awareness about avoiding teen pregnancy, STD's, drugs and alcohol abuse. Theater and art are both good outlets for child victims within their healing processes it is a form of counseling in itself.

Mama's Don't Let Your Babies Grow Up To Be Drunk Boys (Cowboys Are Fine)

Just like a yawn is contagious, Alcoholism is contagious. Parental exposure and peer pressure are key factors. If your child has been exposed to alcohol abuse or neglect seek professional counseling for your child to help repair the psychological and emotional trauma. If you are an adult child of an alcoholic and never received childhood counseling, read books on the topic and seek professional counseling to begin the healing process of the emotional wounds, as early on in life as possible. You'll be glad you did.

Work On Yourself

Focus on your recovery and self-improvement. Make sure your body gets good nutrition, exercise and rest. Do your emotional work. Do your shadow work. Become more aware of your basic human needs. Practice awareness about the effects of alcohol on your body. This chart shows how alcohol interferes with healing processes.

Human Needs	Why It Is A Necessity	Alcohol - Negative Effects
Air	We breath air to oxygenate our body to sustain life.	Alcohol is acidic and causes toxins and carbonic acid that must be exhaled out of the body.
Water	Water is the most cleansing substance on the planet and the substance the body needs most. Over 70% of the body is water.	Alcohol dehydrates the body and increases urination. The body will use up water to neutralize alcohol and rid toxins.

Food	A healthy balanced diet is important as it supplies the body with essential nutrients required to maintain good health and proper function.Some foods provide the amino-acid precursors to neurotransmitters needed to lessen symptoms of withdrawal during recovery	Drinking alcohol adds empty calories, leads to belly fat accumulation and weight gain. Declines physical strength and endurance. Alcohol damages organs.
Exercise Physical Activities	Exercise increases feel good hormones, detoxify the body through sweat, increases metabolism, muscle tone, energy, circulation, and helps prevent adult onset diseases.	Sedentary lifestyle shortens lifespan, alcohol is acidic and drains your physical energy, weakens muscles and promotes weight gain.
Sleep, Rest and Relaxation	Sleep de-stresses and rejuvenates the body. The body repairs itself in the deepest state of sleep. Improves mood and performance.	Alcohol interrupts deep sleep and eventually the body becomes ill. Sleep deprivation has a very bad effect on good health.
Love & Healthy Emotions	Emotional Support & Healthy, Loving Relationships. Giving and receiving love.	Alcohol affects behavior, personality and numbs the emotions and causes damage to relationships.

Sometimes when we go through a trauma we may think it is the end of the world. Usually, you can survive and move on to have a happier life experiences.

Before my divorce I was in beauty and cosmetology. After the trauma of my divorce, I focused on being in a healthy environment and got into healthcare and wellness, I begin to study integrative medicine, alternative medicine, natural medicine, psychology and mind body medicine. I did my shadow-work to find myself and shed light on my shadow side. I had a really bad experience of being married to my first love, my high school sweetheart and watching alcoholism steal him like a body-snatcher and destroy our family.

When Life Gives You Lemons, Make Lemonade

You can grow from every bad experience in life. Something positive can come from negative life experiences. Life is tough sometimes, don't let it make you bitter, let it make you better. I hated prescription drugs and alcohol because these substances were like a body-snatcher that stole my husband but I tried to be understanding to his human condition and tried to see the positive in the experience and turn a bad life experience into a positive psychology perspective. Someday, the experience may allow you to help others. Therefore, I say it was an alcoholic who forced me to take on his responsibilities that made me stronger. It was an alcoholic that hurt my feelings enough to make me invincible to ridicule. It was an alcoholic that forced me into a position that I had to be serious about work ethic for my own survival. It was being miserable living with an alcoholic that made me angry enough to change my own life. It was an alcoholic that put me in the position that I had to give up on him, on us, on our marriage in order to save myself and my daughter. It was an alcoholic that made me begin to demand respect from others. It was an alcoholic that gave me the strength to love myself enough to leave a bad relationship and learn to stand on my own two feet and depend on myself as a single mom at 21 years old.

"If you love someone, let them go, if they come back to you they are yours, if they don't, they never were..."

New Life After Divorce

A year went by, he didn't change and I shifted my focus away from the past and on building a new life and a happier future for my daughter and myself. I worked hard on my issues of independence, studied parenting classes and built a home where my daughter could grown up in a healthier happier environment. We worked with child counselors and I focused on how to be a better parent. I never allowed myself or others to speak badly about her father in front of her, as if you tear down one of the child's parents, it teaches the child not to love that part of themself. I did everything in my power to help her feel safe, secure and balanced so she could heal and grow. I signed her up in swim team and music lessons. I worked in health care and got a college education, became a radiologic technician, physical therapist and chiropractic assistant after a few years I totally transformed my life into a wellness lifestyle became a nutritionist and then I got married again to a friend of mine, a chiropractor who was motivated to make the world a better place through wellness and together we opened the largest chiropractic and wellness clinics in the area, it was a huge success I earned my nutritionist degree and naturopathic doctorate and worked 10 years and we built that location from the ground up with the help of my brothers and we helped many people feel better. I loved my career, and he loved his, we were friends more than spouses because outside of work, our interest were entirely different, so the marriage didn't work out. I loved to travel the world and he was afraid to fly. He loved to hide away in a mountain cabin every weekend. I wanted to take my daughter to explore the world and he wanted to explore hiding away on a secluded lake in the mountains. I didn't want to escape life to the mountains but he found the lady who wanted to do that with him and I found Australia, Europe and the Islands. We had grown as much as we could together, then we grew apart and divorced. I had taught him how to properly manage his business with my business degree and social networking and he had taught me how to be an exceptional leader in the wellness professions. It was a win win for us both and we had very little conflict through the separation it was an uncontested divorce and it never got messy and we are still cordial to one another till this day. Over the next 5 years, I devoted my time to continuous stream of educational seminars all around the world and adding value to the planet though wellness and while helping thousands of patients have healthier lives.

Surviving Alcoholism

10 years flew by since, we survived. Everytime I though she felt stronger and confident then sometimes when we would get news of his condition and life was overshadowed by the fact that his life was still in shambles from alcohol, and then the memories of misery, which I never spoke about with my daughter. We had tried our best to move on beyond the bad experience. My partners and I helped many others heal their lives and health. When I was ready, I branched out and joined a practice in another state. My business was doing great my daughter was a young high-school graduate starting college, too. We were happy and off to a new adventure in California. I began post-graduate studies in anti-aging and functional medicine and during one evening when I was dining alone at a restaurant by the college, a gentleman offered me his menu before the waiter came to assist me, we struck up a conversation and ended up having dinner together. He left the next morning but a long-distance friendship was blossoming, he was from London but lived in Australia where I was coincidentally already signed up to attend a somatic emotional release seminar at the Upledger Institute in Sydney.

For 3 years I frequently traveled and I took my daughter to see other cultures around the world. I made sure my daughter went to private christian schools and had professional support though all of these transitional phases in our lives. I gave my daughter as much love and emotional support that I was capable of. Always careful not to speak badly of her dad, in the home and so not to bring my daughter down. You can never speak badly of a child's parent because the child has 50% of that parents genetics. You want a child to love their parents and that teaches them to love themself. Though I was secretly disappointed because she deserved so much more from him. She never deserved any of that she was the best daughter anyone could have been blessed with. My daughter proved to be resilient, she was deeply into her own life and hobbies, she was active on the swim team. She enjoyed it and won many competitions, she also expressed herself through the arts, she took music and voice lessons. She learn to express herself through her interest in the arts, painting and found her voice through theater. She helped the youth of our community by doing high school peer-pressure awareness skits with the Riverbend players, a mental health outreach community program. It was one of the greatest joys to take her to Shakespeare's globe theater. The greatest joy is watching your children grow and being happy, she learned to speak French and we went to Paris, too. We were both growing and living a better life, it was happy and exciting times but sometimes overshadowed with the sadness and disappointment of her father continually relapsing into alcoholism even after multiple rehab programs. We were finally distanced enough to enjoy our lives without living in a constant state of fear and turmoil. We both worked on our healing processes together, individually and professionally and planned to enroll him in a more whole-person approach rehab in California, some day.

Mental Health and Healthier Relationships

From birth we begin to form our interpersonal relationship skills. If we do not have healthy emotional experiences and good role models, we can develop mental health and relationship issues. A child that has an alcoholic parent can develop adjustment disorders, separation anxiety and self esteem issues from the trauma and neglect of having an alcoholic parent during crucial early childhood development stages. These emotional wounds can cause problems throughout life. It can cause relationship problems and marital problems in their adult life, too. Family counseling is beneficial in helping to heal the old wounds of childhood. There are several helpful books and those that are about how having alcoholic parents during childhood are a good read to prepare you for counseling and offer helpful information to bring awareness to the damaging effects alcoholic parents can have on their children. Unless the child is given professional counseling that can help them through their own healing processes, they will carry the wounds of emotional neglect, trauma and scars with them into every relationship throughout their whole lives.

Alcohol Use When Feeling Unloved

Many drink alcohol as a crutch when they feel they are not receiving or giving enough love. When we fall in love, it is the ultimate joy. The act of making love and making another life is pure joy. Life is about love and relationships and getting to that healthy place of love & joy in our lives and relationships, again. Alcohol is not the drug we need it is love, love is what we seek. During times when we may not be in a satisfying loving relationship it is important to find supportive other people or group therapy instead of turning to alcohol in times of loneliness.

We All Come From A Place Of Love & Joy

Codependency vrs. Counterdependency

Counterdependency is a label for people who refuse emotional attachment. Counter dependency may cause a "flight from intimacy" in your adult relationships. It is not a disease. It is a set of protective adult behaviors caused by unseen and unhealed developmental childhood traumas that happened between the ages of 9 and 36 months, during the toddler stage of development. Your can change these shadow behaviors by healing the underlying emotional traumas that are causing them. Healing counter-dependent behaviors as an adult starts with connecting the dots between what happened to you as a child and what is happening in your adult relationships are interconnected. These behaviors typically involve avoidance of intimacy in your adult relationships by creating rigid boundaries, pushing others away, appearing overly independent, and by acting strong, blaming others and keeping very busy, too busy for intimacy.

"The codependent person will be attracted to the only alcoholic in a lineup of 100 people".

Line up 100 people who all look the same, 99 of them are non-drinkers, only 1 is an alcoholic and subconsciously, the codependent will be attracted to and choose the 1 and only alcoholic in the group. If you find yourself always ending up in relationships with an addict or alcoholic, you may be codependent, like I was. Doing some shadow work counseling may help. My 3 year, long-distance engagement ended after his bachelor party. Apparently, he had gotten drunk and made the bad decision to sleep with the stripper, after I found glitter and bobby pins all over the bedroom, his explanation was that he was drinking and he believed that a man could be totally and completely in love with someone but have sex with someone else, just for sex and I said, "yes" you can be in love with someone and have sex with someone else, but that someone, is not going to be me, and I immediately ended our engagement. He was already blaming alcohol for his mistakes and expecting me to forgive him for sex outside of our relationship. I wasn't going down that road again.

Oh, No! Not Again!!!

I was finished being the co dependent in life. I disconnected and flipped polar opposite. Why do we disconnect? We disconnect because we have been hurt in the past. By disconnecting, we think we will never be hurt again, but that is a lonely existence. None of us come into this life alone, none of us will get through this life alone. Life is about love and relationships and getting to that place of love and joy in our lives and relationships. Refusing to need other people or by denying that you or they have any needs in the first place and avoiding intimate situations as often as possible is called counterdependency.

The key in understanding counter-dependency is differentiating it from healthy autonomy. Healthy autonomy is a state of confident self-reliance in which an individual

a) recognizes their interdependency with others;
b) has a sense of controlling their own destiny and
c) is not unduly controlled or influenced by others.

On the surface, counter-dependency may look similar to a healthy autonomy. For example, both involve the capacity to separate from others. But what drives counter-dependency is an "avoidance mindset," namely the avoidance of relying on others because of a fundamental mistrust of the consequence of doing so. In addition, although these individuals might have superficially positive relationships, but because they fundamentally fear intimacy and do not trust others, they do not form lasting deep relationships. Indeed, even in marriage, a counter dependent will hide core aspects of their experience, resist showing dependency needs, and be reluctant to open up. Instead, they will often offer a superficial confidence and/or simply separate and avoid whenever a need or opportunity for deep emotional connection surfaces. It can be a very frustrating experience for the partner.

One of the key definitions of counter-dependency is the person has an unhealthy resistance of having a reliance on others, in any way. To understand what counter-dependency we must first understand co-dependency, which is a mental state where the person has trouble differentiating their autonomy from persons close to them. In healthy autonomy, everyone is an individual with respected healthy boundaries but are able to be self-supporting and have healthy interpersonal relationships but is capable of depending on each other when appropriate. Healthy autonomy is a state of confident self-reliance in which an individual

- can recognize their interdependence with other individuals;
- a healthy agentic sense of self-empowerment and a sense they can control their own destiny
- the person can consider others opinions but can make their own decisions and they are not typically, controlled or overly influenced by others.

However, initially, upon observing a counter-dependent personality type, it may appear to be similar to a healthy autonomy. For example, healthy autonomy and counter-dependency both, involve the capacity to separate from others and what will drive a counter-dependent is their "avoidance mindset." They will avoid relying on other people because somewhere in their development an emotional trauma or injury occurred, someone betrayed them or hurt them deeply in some way and thereafter they developed a mistrust of people, this mistrust carries over into every future relationship, where the other person will always have to prove themselves trustworthy, and often on an ongoing continual basis. No matter what you do to earn a counter dependants trust, it will not be good enough, and in fact, you will likely never earn it, until the counter dependant gets into therapy or does their emotional healing work. Additionally, if these individuals appear to have positive relationships, fundamentally they fear intimacy and do not trust others. Counter-dependants do not form lasting deep relationships. Even in marriage, it is a counter-dependent trait to hide information from their partners, important core aspects of their feelings, you never know how the counter-dependant really feels, because they won't give their partners any ammo to use against them later because their deepest fear is to be hurt, again. They often view love as war and they are experts at covert avoidance, they would rather avoid and abandon than to submit themselves to the risk of feeling pain from opening themselves up or being vulnerable, in any way. They run from relationship intimacy. They resist showing that they need anyone, and they are reluctant to open up. Instead, they offer superficial intimacy, and exude superficial confidence and frequently separate or break-up and avoid their own need or sabotage any opportunity for a deep emotional love connection. It is a very frustrating type of relationship experience for those who try to become their partner.

Signs Of Being A Counterdependent:

- Your moto is depend on no one because you trust no one
- You were badly hurt by someone you loved at an early age and you vowed to never love someone and get hurt like that ever again
- You felt betrayed by a loved one, and you swore to never trust again
- You vowed to never let anyone have power to hurt you again
- You suffer anxiety in close intimate relationships because you want to open up and be vulnerable but the old trust issues won't allow you
- You have a brick wall around your heart
- You won't let love in, you have a subconscious block
- You lack trust in others and you are suspicious of ulterior motives
- You suspect authentic kindness and you fear being manipulated
- Love cannot penetrate through your brick wall nor hurt you, again
- You hide your insecurities from others
- You show little awareness for the needs and wants of others
- You may tend to sexualise any touch or on the flip you are asexual
- You like to always look good and be 'right'
- You often exhibit perfectionist behaviours.
- You are afraid to appear weak or to loose control
- You have to be the one in control
- You are cut off from your real self and real feelings
- You rarely ask for help because you won't let yourself need anyone
- You are often lonely from shutting others out
- Your conflicted between being lonely and needing alone time
- You need alone time to recover from being exhausted by fighting constantly to keep people shut out of your life
- You don't welcome friends into your personal space freely
- You meet your friends in their environment so you can flee at will
- You constantly struggling to keep others from getting too close
- You want a lover and friends but you keep them at a safe distance.
- You refuse to open all the way up to your friends, family or lover
- You never allow them the opportunity to disappoint you.
- You keep even your closest relationships pushed away at arms length, never really letting anyone close to or close into your heart.

Often, recovering codependent people flip into counterdependency, which is equally unhealthy. Opposites attract subconsciously, perhaps to try to fix something that is broken inside of themselves that they recognize is broken in the other person, too. A codependent person will inevitably choose a counterdependent person and vice versa, to form an emotional rollercoaster love relationships, resulting in a vicious cycle of perpetually repelling each others shadow sides, reinforcing the negative cycle and perpetually forming painful and unhealthy interpersonal skills and patterns. The counterdependant/codependent couple can potentially survive if they do their shadow work on their own individually and then together in family counseling, otherwise, the relationship dynamic is doomed. If the codependent finally gathers the strength to try and walk away from the emotionally aloof counterdependent the relationship will likely end. The attraction is that their subconscious mind recognizes an unresolved issue with a parent, from a childhood wounding, and they want their lover to bring this unresolved childhood wound out from the subconscious so they have a chance to heal the emotional wound in adulthood, however painful it may be. They both feel victimized from childhood but wrongfully blame each other for the pain. The dysfunctional duo destroys themselves and each other if they do not do their shadow work through the unhealthy behaviors together to break the pattern, and until they do their shadow work they will never win love from each other, or understand each other and their relationship will likely end in divorce. However, the pattern sometimes totally switches! The once counterdependent panics and gets clingy, trying to hold on to the formerly codependent person who now might become cold and shut down, in other words, counterdependent. Basically, counseling is good for everyone.

Heartbroken & Self-Medicating

Alcohol has long been used as a break-up remedy for a reason. Anyone going through a divorce can tell you about heartache and pain of falling out of love with a lover. Alcohol is numbing but it is never going to heal your broken heart. Alcohol numbs people's feelings and heartaches, but only temporarily. Many are using Alcohol to numb feelings that they don't want to feel or deal with. It's one thing to drown your sorrows for an evening when you lose your lover or job. Getting drunk is a poor method of coping and your problems will still be there the next day.

Drinking Alcohol Never Solved Anyone's Problems

You can't use alcohol to cope with your feelings and emotions, very long. It doesn't fix the problem permanently nor does it change how you feel for very long it only prolongs the problem and allows time to procrastinate in resolving issues. Using alcohol to mask for negative emotions leaves the pressure of emotions building up inside and when they surface it will be like a pressure cooker exploding. Drinking progresses into developing a habit. Trying to drink your problems away wont work and is only going to cause you bigger problems later, knowing that the alcohol habit is progressive it is a habit that leads to dependance, alcohol abuse and alcoholism. If you drink long enough, you begin to think like an alcoholic. Drink longer you will begin to act like an alcoholic, keep on drinking and you will become and alcoholic. Like attracts like. Like minded people, think alike and act alike. Surround yourself with enough users and your in the alcohol trap and it is a hard mess to clean up and get out of without a lot of pain and suffering.

Drinking Problems Away

Problems are a part of life that are meant to be dealt with in a healthy and proactive way. Problems are not supposed to be washed down inside by guzzling alcohol. Eventually, all suppressed emotions and problems will come to a head, like an explosive volcano. Read books, confide in a mentor or seek help from a professional counselor. Talk your issues out, don't procrastinate. As easy as it is to drink away your problems, you are only sabotaging yourself by pouring a depressant into an already sad and unhappy brain so alcohol doesn't solve anything. After self-medicating with alcohol and you wake up, you will only feel worse, and on top of the problem that is still there, you'll have a hangover, too.

You can never drink your problems away, and you will end up with a real drinking problem if you think you are drinking away your problems, you are only creating more problems. The only solution is to face your problems. Deal with your problems with a clear head and deal with your problems without involving alcohol to the problem-solving process. Some of the worst problem solving ideas were thought of while people were drinking alcohol. After you sober up, usually, you can clearly see your drunk ideas are quite a bit of nonsense that will not solve your problem and was a waste of time and mental energy to ever be in a drunken state when trying to problem solve. Asking your drunk buddies for advice is not such a good idea either. Never ask advice from someone you wouldn't switch places with in life. If you do, you will get drunk shitty advice which is even worse than regular shitty advice.

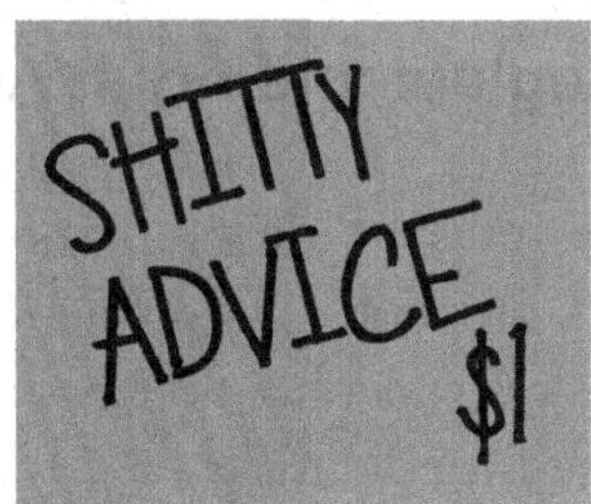

Growing Up on Alcohol

Children are very influential. Children soak up patterns and behaviors like a sponge. Many people don't even know why they drink. It's good to look at your earliest memories regarding alcohol so you understand what drives or triggers you to drink. Up until I quit drinking wine, all of my closest friends, with the exception of a few people, were all drinkers, usually, wine drinkers. Most all of my family, role-models and teachers were drinkers at some point in their lives, all except my mother and grandmother. Therefore, one may say Alcohol consumption can be learned and may even be considered contagious. Especially, to teen children. Peer pressure prevention is a big factor to consider in effective prevention programs.

Peer Pressure in Late Teen Children

There has been at least one university hazing death each year from 1969 to 2017. 82% percent of deaths from hazing involve alcohol. In fact, alcohol poisoning is the most common cause of death. The majority of these deaths are age 18-21. Children who come from strict homes where parents not only have negative attitudes about drinking but also monitor their children's academic progress and other activities also have less risk for alcoholism and drugs. Children who attend religious services frequently, and are taught to believe that religion is important in their lives have lower rates of chemical abuse. One study showed abuse at about 7% for religious teens and 17% for non-religious.

Babies & Children of Alcohol

The saddest thing in our culture of alcoholism are the babies born with alcohol fetal syndrome. The effects on children are catastrophic. An estimated 40,000 newborns each year are affected by FAS, Fetal Alcohol Syndrome from being exposed to alcohol before birth. Developing babies lack the ability to process alcohol with their liver, which is not fully formed. They absorb all of the alcohol and have the same blood alcohol content as the mother. Alcohol causes more harm than heroin or cocaine during pregnancy. The Institute of Medicine says, "Of all the substances of abuse alcohol produces by far the most serious neurobehavioral effects in the fetus."

Childhood Abuse and Neglect and Adult Alcohol Abuse

Children of alcoholic parents tend to develop more personality disorders than children of parents who don't drink alcohol. Researchers indicate victims of child abuse and neglect may be at increased risk for alcohol abuse during adult-hood. Thus, alcohol serves as a poor coping means for self-medicating

- Mechanism to cope and escape the trauma of abuse of alcoholic parent
- Childhood victimization and the related depression
- A way to reduce feelings of isolation and loneliness
- Self-medication in an attempt to gain control over the experience
- A way to temporarily feel better self-esteem
- A form of self-destructive behavior

Accordingly, factors such as poor coping skills, antisocial behavior, and abuse-related post traumatic stress disorder (PTSD) may help mediate the relationship between childhood victimization and adult alcohol problems.

Children and Elderly Alcoholic Caregivers

Being a caregiver is one of the most selfless roles anyone can fulfill. It means putting someone else's needs above your own giving your time, patience and understanding. It can create a sense of purpose, but it can burdensome and emotional and psychologically trying, especially if the care involves a terminal condition and if no other person shares the load. Whether the role consists of providing care for a problem child, a cancer patient or an ill, disabled or elderly person, the demands can drive many caregivers to use and abuse substances to cope. Widowed and elderly are the age group with the most alcoholism, feeling let down, disappointed and depressed over the loss of their spouse and many families will leave their infant and young children with their grandparents or great grandparents which many not be the best idea, especially if they are drinkers or substance abusers. Children are most influenced by alcoholic caregivers, its a bad example and not worth the risk, additionally, it's not fair to the elderly to be mistreated by frazzled substance abusing end of life caregivers, either. Please, do a thorough background check of all your loved ones caregivers, it is not worth the risk as psychological abuse cause permanent emotional damage to children and elderly victims.

Post Divorce Life

It was because of alcohol that we were never able to have a stable family environment nor provide that happy loving attentive family foundation that helps children be strong and confident. The best gift you can give children is an alcohol free, happy, stable two parent home. It was a disappointment, and I had to do my best as a single parent to provide my child a stable happy home. I had to be the mom and the dad. Alcohol is one of the main reasons that we have an epidemic of single parent homes in America. Once my daughter graduated high school, we decided to move across country to California when a college opportunity came up for her. We packed our bags and started a whole new chapter in life. The difficulties of moving across country to L.A. proved to be challenging. California has a way of making people find themselves, if there are past emotional wounds, they will surface in LA, because all your buttons will be pushed in the city's hectic environment. It is a great place to work on yourself because there are many self-improvement classes, counselors and family therapist options available. There are so many people living in one city, living there teaches you to connect to your community family in a large way. There are so many people, so much traffic, so much waiting in long lines to do everything, it test your patience, it test your compassion for your fellow man. Instead of road rage and being angry for being stalled in massive traffic jams and waiting in line for 2 hours to get your license or waiting in line an hour just to buy a hot dog. LA will teach you patience. The rest of the world thinks it is a crazy rat race they would never choose to live in. I chose to live in this city, this chaos, this is my town, these are my people. I love L.A. it is like the whole world is crammed into one city, there are people from every state in the U.S. and it is a smorgasbord of cultures, in a good way. There are a lot of people with great success stories and there are a lot of heart broken people with heart breaking stories of loss. If you look into the histories of many celebrities, they suffered some childhood trauma, which makes them better actors or entertainers because as a child many of them learned early on, how to make an emotionally distraught or substance abusing parents laugh or change a negative mood, comedy is an art of taking life's tragedies and turning them into a comedy. Laughter is always the best medicine. You can only laugh it off for so long and mental illness and alcoholism are not a laughing matter. LA is a city with extreme stresses and extreme successes and I love it more than anywhere I've been on the planet. Many children of alcohol abuse have some form of emotional trauma issues or developmental trauma. Awareness is the first step to health and well being.

The Shadow-Self Childhood Trauma Subconscious Addiction Risk

According to Jungian psychology, as we grow up, we all will have a "childhood wounding". We all have a wounded inner child that needs love and support. Spouses and children of abusive alcoholics often suffer from emotional syndromes ranging from codependency to counter-dependency. Being betrayed by a friend or a family member is one of the worst feelings ever. Some children are polyvictimized, they have suffered more than one form of wounding or maltreatment. Children shut down when they have an emotional wounding and their shadow self is born. Children make self-protection contracts to protect themselves to never allow anyone to hurt or harm them again, this is known as the "childhood wounding" allowing the birth of the "shadow-self". I believe doing your shadow work can help in overcoming many emotional wounds caused by childhood traumas or abusive caregivers. There are many books on the shadow self that are helpful. Some believe it is best to do this work with a counselor, especially if you were a victim of child abuse in any form. If you were, your not alone and its important to work through those emotional traumas, wounds and scars with a counselor. I agree.

Childhood Abuse and Neglect and Adult Alcohol Abuse

Nearly 700,000 children are abused in the U.S annually and in the generations before it use to be much worse, the baby boomer generation and prior generations it was customary to whip their children as physical punishment or verbally abuse and traumatise their children by yelling at them and making them wear a dunce hat in school. Inhumane cruelty is a precursor to alcoholism and a side effect, as well. Researchers have proposed several hypotheses as to why victims of child abuse and neglect may be at increased risk for alcohol abuse during adulthood. Thus, alcohol may serve as the following:

- A mechanism to cope with or escape from the trauma of childhood victimization and the related depression
- A way to reduce feelings of isolation and loneliness
- Self-medication in an attempt to gain control over the experience
- A way to improve self-esteem
- A form of self-destructive behavior.

Accordingly, factors such as poor coping skills, antisocial behavior, and abuse-related posttraumatic stress disorder (PTSD) may help mediate the relationship between childhood victimization and adult alcohol problems.

Researchers have suggested that for some victims of childhood abuse, alcohol may serve as a coping mechanism to deal with the trauma associated with the abuse and its detrimental consequences.

Which Came 1st, The Chicken Or The Egg

Researchers have studied alcohol abuse as both a contributor to and a consequence of child abuse. The dilemma was which came first, does alcohol cause parents to commit child abuse or does child abuse cause alcoholism later on in adulthood. The answer is both. Several studies have indicated that parental alcohol abuse may increase a child's risk of experiencing abuse or neglect by another person at some point in life. Studies found that women who had experienced childhood maltreatment were more likely to have alcohol problems as adults than other women. Alcohol use as a coping mechanism has been identified as a mediator between childhood abuse and neglect and subsequent alcohol problems. Therapy intervention is proven to help those victims develop more positive coping mechanisms.

Juveniles And Alcohol

Among juvenile inmate populations, in teens that commit crimes, 80 percent have a history of abusing drugs or alcohol. The percentages are the same as adult offenders, which shows that the problematic association between criminal behavior and drinking tends to develop early in life. Alcohol is a killer that ruins and ends lives. Pre-adults with their hormones raging combined with alcohol is a disaster waiting to happen. According to the CDC, Excessive drinking is responsible for more than 4,300 deaths among underage youth each year, and cost the U.S. more than $24 billion in economic costs. Although drinking by persons under the age of 21 is illegal, people aged 12 to 20 years drink 11% of all alcohol consumed in the United States.

High School to College Passage Class Trip

According to the U.S. National Institute on Alcohol Abuse and Alcoholism (NIAAA) approximately 1,825 college students between the ages of 18 and 24 die each academic year from accidental alcohol related injuries. Students celebrate their successful passing of high school or graduating up to the next level of college. During spring break, 44 % of college girls and 75 % of college boys drink and get drunk every day of their trip. Approximately 50% of college students binge drink and many will drink to the point of passing out at least once during their vacation and some of them die from alcohol poisoning. For many, class trips turn into a time of alcohol-related incidents including alcohol poisoning, car wrecks, boat, jet ski accidents, drownings, assaults, rapes and unprotected sex. All of these situations can have life-long altering consequences. Spring break should be the passage from adolescence into responsible young adulthood and that should be emphasized by shapperones and school faculty that it is not a vacation for everybody in class to get drunk together.

People Most Sensitive To Alcohol

Some groups of people are likely to be affected more by alcohol and should be more careful of their level of drinking on any one occasion:

- young adults
- older people
- those with low body weight
- those with other health problems
- those on medicines or other drugs

As well as the risk of accident and injury, drinking alcohol regularly is linked to long term risks such as heart disease, cancer, liver disease, and epilepsy.

High Risk Housewives & Women

Alcohol use by women is a growing public health problem in the United States. Alcohol use has been glamorized by reality TV shows, especially where I live, in Beverly Hills and in other larger cities across the U.S. Additionally, women are being targeted with marketing and ad campaigns customized to attract women drinkers and it is showing in the statistics. Some wine manufacturers even name wines a name pertaining exclusively to women on their label and many offer Mother's Day promotions to encourage moms to drink to cope with the stresses of motherhood. In the U.S., alcohol has become the most common mother's little helper according to studies with 70% of Caucation women are drinkers, 47% of African American women, 41% of Hispanic, and 37% Asian women are likely to drink alcohol and the death rates reflect the problem as the rate of alcohol-related deaths for women ages 35 to 54 has more than doubled since 1999 in the United States with a high number of deaths from liver disease.

Pregnancy Alcohol Risk

If you are pregnant or planning a pregnancy, the safest approach is not to drink alcohol at all, to keep risks to your baby to a minimum. That is why planned parenthood is so important. It is best not to drink at least 3 months prior to your pregnancy and abstain through pregnancy and breast feeding.

- Drinking during pregnancy can lead to long-term harm to the baby, with the more you drink, the greater the risk.
- Most women either do not drink alcohol (19%) or stop drinking during pregnancy (40%).
- The risk of harm to the baby is likely to be low if a woman has drunk only small amounts of alcohol before she knew she was pregnant or during pregnancy.
- Slow or restricted growth
- facial abnormalities
- learning and behavioral disorders, which are long lasting and may be lifelong

Women who find out they became pregnant, accidentally, after already having drank alcohol during conception and early pregnancy, should avoid further drinking, but should be aware that it is possible but unlikely, in most cases, that their baby has been affected. Drinking after missing your period, during your pregnancy effects on your baby includes physical, mental and behaviour problems including learning disabilities which can have lifelong implications. The risk of such problems are likely to be greater the more you drink. If you are worried about how much you have been drinking before you found out you are pregnant inform your OBGYN doctor immediately. Additionally, have your baby in a hospital that has a neo-natal intensive care units available.

My New Life Of Stress And The Building Alcohol Tolerance Inside

I was super fit working out everyday, writing a wellness book, "The Balance Diet and Lifestyle", when I moved from a smaller city of 450,000, to a city of 20+ million. I was immersed in a whole new culture, of health freaks, and I was one, too. It was a world of exciting new opportunities. It was an exciting move but I did suffer from culture shock. Hollywood is a party town and I came from the bible belt.

Since my career is in health and beauty, it was a refreshing change as LA is filled with the health conscious and there are plenty of people that are always seeking to look and feel better, my area of healthcare expertise. Within a few weeks of arriving in LA I was working in one of the most prestigious clinics in Beverly Hills caring for highly ambitious people, celebrities, actors and models who take their health and appearance seriously, they spend fortunes in treatments to help themselves look and feel their best with everything from plastic surgery, beauty treatments and various other multiple disciplinary wellness treatment clinics. Within 3 months I was on MTV and have been on several TV shows over the first 10 years in LA.

All of the health clinics I worked in, prior to owning my own clinic, all catered to celebrities and the people behind the scenes who really run the show, as well as the general public. The first clinic was low profile, with private entrance for celebrities catered to celebrities for over 35 years in Beverly Hills. Celebrities are just like the rest of us, they also have the same basic needs but their healthcare can be more crucial as they usually have higher stress levels due to their demanding schedules and constant public scrutiny. They often have more opportunities and temptations for fall into a pattern of alcohol and substance abuse, than the rest of us. We tend to think a celebrities life is all fun and games, it is a hard working life and they get physically exhausted working on set all through the night or performing 4 hour long concerts while on tour, nightly for 3 months not to mention the jet lag of travel to boot but the show must go on night after night. They may be in NYC tonight, the next night in Los Angeles, the next night in Sydney, the next night in London. Celebrities work hard and many use substances to get them through. Their body's need super nutrition, IV vitamin drips and power naps but many resort to pills and booze and sadly, those are the ones that end up dead.

California is filled with extremes, the most health conscious people in the U.S. and on the flip the highest in drug and alcohol abuse in the country. There is a gym, pilates or yoga studio on every corner, and there is no shortage of wellness clients. After a long day at work the yoga classes did not seem like enough to calm my mind and body from the stress of surviving in one of the world's most expensive cities. My career became my most important focus. I became a workaholic. Many work-a-holics become alcoholics. It starts from having poor coping skills then progresses into self-medicating stress with alcohol. Many white collar workers are vulnerable to alcohol abuse. Stock brokers responsible for the losses of many retirement funds who also lost their jobs during the stock market crash, also became addicts and alcoholics, and some actually committed suicide from having poor coping skills. When you play big, you lose big. Many stressful situations are enough to drive people to drink.

Drinking Alcohol Kills Your Motivation

LA Woman

Balance is important to your recovery and to successful sober living. If you find your stress level is too much, make a move, your not a tree. Sometimes we have to take a step back and pace our lifestyle to match our coping skills. I remember, the most difficult thing to adapt to was noise pollution. I remember going into the interior bathroom to get away from the sound of traffic, for a quiet moment. I also remember having to drink a glass of wine and wearing ear plugs to block out the noise of the LA freeways to get to sleep at night before I moved from downtown to Beverly Hills. It takes a while to get accustomed to all the noise and that is an irritating stress of its own in LA because there are 20+ million cars constantly whizzing up and down the freeways of southern California and the sound was audible from the homes my daughter and I lived in for the first ten years. I worked in a clinic that serviced Hollywood A-listers for 35 years and I worked there several years. I worked as a spokesperson for a beauty aesthetics equipment company traveling all over the U.S. to tradeshows and healthcare conventions and loved it but it was an exhausting commitment that robbed my own life of balance. Then, I was approached and offered a position by one of the most famous plastic surgery groups in LA as their bariatric aftercare and weight loss director. Many of our doctors, there, were featured on shows such as the Swan and the Doctors. I was the weight loss director of 11 clinics in southern California there were alot of promotional events, parties, seminars, trade shows. Additionally, I was a spokesperson for the company, so I had to travel to attend most of the events that we sponsored throughout southern California. I worked that position for several years until I was noticed and offered a position by one of our nation's top advisors to 4 U.S. Presidents, he hired me to join his corporate team as his wellness director and assistant medical director of a chain of integrative medical clinics. Simultaneously, I was continuing postgraduate studies in Mind Body Medicine at Harvard medical school. Behind the scenes, after the long work days, I was exercising less and was lonely and I was starting to drink wine. The friends I had and the man I dated was more sophisticated, more cultured and they were wine fanatics.

There was a four year period, I was also doing community volunteer work, I was an executive board member of the chamber of commerce, I was the Ambassador committee chairperson, overseeing a group of 50+ fellow ambassadors and making sure every new business in town had a smashing grand opening ceremony. I was working with the Mayors and also lobbying at the state capital and our nation's capital, in Washington, DC in support of integrative healthcare benefits and insurance coverage for the greater good of the U.S. healthcare system. At all those thousands of business mixers and it became a customary part of the networking lifestyle to enjoy a glass of wine and talk to fellow business owners, politicians and lobbyist at these promotional events. I once asked a fellow physician colleague if he could write me a letter of recommendation for enrollment into a post graduate program and he wrote, "Dr. Peters can accomplish more in a short amount of time than anyone I've ever known". I was a textbook case of being on the road to becoming a highly functioning wino.

The Wine Lie

The wine industry began ramping up in 2008, and pumping up Americans to drink wine for the health benefits of Resveratrol. Many resveratrol campaigns came out by the wine industry, it was a media frenzy, even on a 60 Minutes broadcast, Barbara Walters was raving about the anti-aging and antioxidant benefits of resveratrol, and yes, it is a great benefit to our health, but having alcohol as a source is not. It was all over the media, a daily glass of wine is good for anti-aging and then we all had an excuse to make our wine drinking justifiable. The wine industry sales campaigns are strong and persistent in California. Grapes are one of California's best gross product sellers and then to top it all off major universities came out with studies saying that drinking 1 glass of wine per day for women and 2 glasses a day for men would greatly benefit your health for the antioxidant content and for anti-aging benefits of Resveratrol.

Wine Zaps Your Energy & Leaves You Depressed The Next Day

We were all getting aboard this trainwreck of daily wine consumption and what they were not telling the public is that the grape crops are tainted with chemical residues that are hazardous to our health. According to the World Health Organization (WHO) despite studies linking moderate alcohol consumption to heart health, picking up a glass of wine isn't the answer to prolonged life. The health risks associated with alcohol consumption, like liver disease, heavily outweigh the slight benefits of drinking wine, especially since those same heart healthy benefits can be achieved through diet and exercise. Yet people all over the world are still consuming high levels of alcohol.

Additionally, alcohol in fact acts on the same receptor sites in the brain that GABA (Gamma-Aminobutyric Acid) does. Remember GABA, it is a non-protein amino acid that functions as a neurotransmitter, that all alcoholic beverages, including wine block neural pathways along with blocking most of the other neurotransmitters that are important in sending signals around your brain and regulating bodily functions. The ads also fail to give informed consent that alcohol also negatively affects organs and negatively affects all your bodily systems. GABA is more important for anti-aging than resveratrol, as it also increases HGH levels by improving your sleep, since your night-time growth hormone release is linked to sleep quality and depth and the growth hormone you produce in your sleep also repairs damage to the body. Alcohol disrupts this important phase of reparative sleep.

Alcohol Beauty Destroyer

Alcohol dehydrates your body and skin and may even result in wrinkles and cause the appearance of early aging. The effects of alcohol accelerates signs of aging and includes, premature wrinkles, dryness, collagen loss, reduced volume, loss of elasticity, redness and broken blood vessels and sagging in your skin. The more you drink the more quickly aging progresses. Alcohol is acidic negatively changes body chemistry and damages DNA. If you are a drinker the best thing you can do to slow down aging quick drinking alcohol and switch to ionized water and fresh juices and herbal teas. You will get more antioxidants than you get with wine and you will preserve your youthful beauty longer without the destroying effects of alcohol.

Alcohol in America

Every generation of America has had its era of use and alcohol issues. Even though we are in the midst of an Alcohol epidemic, the issue with alcohol is nothing new in America, from the beginning till the end of prohibition, alcohol consumption was never quit it just made the black market and bootleggers rich. The roaring 30's had real cocaine in cola. The 60's had a hippy drug use culture. The baby-boomer generation was sold on an over indulgent lifestyle of beach-goers wasting away in Margaritaville. Generation-X sold on sex and drugs & rock-n-roll. The Generation XYZ Rave's heavy alcohol use and ecstasy. The Millenials are being sold on EDM music party generation of millenials with designer drugs and copious amounts of alcohol.

Working Class Quick Fix

Stress grows into a silent killer of the working class, think of the blue collar working punching a time clock, from sunrise to sunset in our factories, or the single mom working a 2nd job struggling to make ends meet, or the farmer whose crops failed last season and the bank is foreclosing on his land, and the stockbroker who lost everything when the stock market crashed. When we work all day and get off work late, we spent the day chasing dollars, instead of doing what we really wanted to do, but there is a happy hour in every restaurant on every corner waiting for 5:00 to tick by. You can easily fall into a habit of stopping for a quick pick-me-up and then progressing into staying well past happy hour at the bar, or the housewife that is having a glass or two of wine with dinner a couple of times a week. People also use alcohol as a crutch for dealing with all kinds of "problems, be it stress, boredom or family and relationship problems. Happy hours were created for the working class. That's what the term "happy hour" means, it's an hour to get happy drinking before going home and facing issues there. Alcohol is not the solution.

City Life = Added Stress

In larger cities, there are so many options and opportunities along with that comes temptation, when there are multiple parties every night where the wine and champagne flows and as from my experience, I never did drugs, so it takes true inner strength to hold on to your health values in a city of so many opportunities for parties and over-indulgence and extreme stress. Just driving is a nerve wrecking experience and for several years I was driving a 4 hour round trip commute a day commuting to our 11 plastic surgery clinics as a director by the time I got home I thought I needed a glass of wine to calm down from the stress of avoiding hundreds of near-miss automobile accidents, and if you live and drive in LA this is a daily experience. Everyone drives in LA, there are 20 million people trying to share a couple of freeways and it can take an hour to go 5 miles by the time I would get home at night a glass of wine was a welcomed relaxant.

Demographic Access & Conditioning

California is wine country. Wine is big business and part of the Californian lifestyle is drinking the wine we produce. The industry promotes a heavy presence of being a part of the California lifestyle. Even, though I knew better, I began to drink the wine regularly, anyway. Healthwise, it seemed we all fell for the ad campaigns, to drink wine for the Resveratrol and antioxidants for anti-aging which is better if we take it in a vitamin supplement form without the negative health effects of drinking alcohol. I knew alcohol wasn't the best stress coping option. I couldn't take enough vacations to deal with the amount of stress I had so I justified my wine drinking as being a better habit than taking a pain reliever or prescription anti-depressants. In hindsight, I knew, we can get resveratrol in a pill without the damaging effects of alcohol. I used wine to self-medicate my high stress lifestyle. When I drank wine, I felt no physical pain. It did not make me drunk because I did it in small amounts over a long period of time in moderation, which is typically how a tolerance is built up over time. However, there were always negative side effects, I suffered from heart-burn which was from the acidity of the wine and the sugar overload. I would snack on other healthy foods such as nuts and berries, but alcohol makes us want to snack more than usual so we end up taking in more calories which lead to weight issues. Being overweight and obesity lead to other serious health conditions and co-morbities associated with obesity.

In LA, there are over 6 million new residents moving into LA every year and just as many people leave LA. I have met and made so many wonderful friends from all around the world in LA. Many people are transplants, and it seems it is part of the LA culture that everyone has an extended family in LA and it's sad when the move away. In the days before skype and snapchat, the odds were great that the people you make friends in LA may end up leaving and going back to wherever they come from and you never see them again. I got depressed over the loss of a few friends leaving and going back to foreign countries where they were originally from, I visited some abroad, but then there are those you never hear from or see ever again. I numbed my emotions many times over the loss of friends and family with wine.

The Loss of a Loved One is a Trigger for all Drinkers. Drinking Numbs Emotions

Older Americans Drink To Numb

We all go through phases throughout life. After mid-life, many people drink to numb feelings of loneliness. After the children are grown, we are alone more and many suffer empty nest syndrome and drink out of loneliness. Many lose a spouse and suffer depression and self-medicate with alcohol. Life is full of changes but there is a healthy solution for every phase without alcohol. It is entirely possible that the consumption of alcohol is to blame for the increase of adult onset diseases that baby boomers are now suffering with in mid life. A 2017 study shows that alcohol abuse in women increased 83.7 % and this is a sign of the aging Baby Boomers hitting the bottle too hard and men 65 and older went up a whopping 106.7 %.

According to a recently published study in the Journal of the American Medical Association:

- The number of adults 65 years and older who drank has risen higher than the national average.
- The average number of adults 65 and older suffering from alcohol abuse had risen by nearly 107 %.

The National Council on Alcoholism and Drug Dependence shows that:

- Alcohol-related problems are the cause of 14 % of senior emergency room admissions
- Alcohol use causes 20 % of elderly psychiatric hospital admissions.
- The majority of Baby Boomers are struggling with alcoholism.
- Elderly adults are hospitalized as often for alcohol-related problems as they are for heart attacks.
- Approximately, 50 % of nursing home residents have alcohol use disorders.

All of these statistics raise the questions of why this is happening to our seniors and is a real danger that has gone unnoticed until it is a big problem.

AGING AND ALCOHOL ABUSE

Some of the more obvious reasons for alcohol misuse among older adults include physical pains and other health problems. However, one major cause linked to the emergence of alcohol abuse among seniors is as a form of self-medication against feelings of depression or anxiety. Studies show that currently, as many as 1 in 4 seniors have a mental illness and that the estimated total number of older adults struggling with mental health disorders is expected to reach 15 million by 2030. If an individual was not dealing with these mental health issues before, they can be and frequently are triggered by environmental factors such as facing a newly empty nest or a loss of purpose that can accompany retirement. While the average transition time from what could be considered regular alcohol use to alcoholism can take years, seniors are much more vulnerable to rapid, dramatic changes in their drinking habits triggered by these sudden, significant changes in their daily routine.

One reason why Baby Boomers may choose to turn to alcohol rather than professional help is due to having lived the majority of their lives during a time when there was a much stronger stigma against mental illness. Some may find it easier or less embarrassing to cope privately with alcohol, despite the obvious dangers.

Elderly Alcoholism

Alcoholism has been called the widow-maker. Binge drinking raises the risk of a heart attack by 70% Drinking causes marital problems, people are more argumentative while drinking and the other negative emotions associated with them. A study completed at Duke University That surveyed 11,000 people over the age of 50 found an extremely high prevalence of binge drinkers and also found a correlation between those who engaged in binge drinking being separated, divorced, or widowed. Binge drinking raises the risk divorce and death in older adults. Alcohol-related emergency room discharges among the elderly reached nearly three-quarters of a million in 2012 The National Council on Alcoholism and Drug Dependence (NCADD) recently reported that widowers over the age of 75 have the highest rate of alcoholism.

ALCOHOL ADDS ADDITIONAL DANGERS FOR SENIORS

Alcohol use disorders can cause a whole host of health problems at any age, they pose even more danger to seniors, mostly due to changes in how the body handles alcohol with age. While someone may have had the same drinking habits for years, their body may no longer be able to keep up with them, making seniors especially at risk for unintentional over-drinking and the potential for accidents such as falls and fractures that come with it. Women, in particular, become more sensitive to the effects of alcohol with age. Heavy drinking can also severely worsen health problems that are common in older adults such as:

- High blood pressure
- Liver problems
- Diabetes
- Osteoporosis
- Memory problems
- Heart problems

Alcohol's negative interactions with various over-counter-medications such as aspirin, acetaminophen, cough syrup, and various pain medications are also magnified in older adults and have a much higher risk of being fatal. Additionally, alcohol lessens motor skills and falls are already one of the highest risk and causes of death in the elderly. Elderly drinkers do not have the metabolism of their youth and can literally get falling down drunk and easily fall down and break a leg or a hip. A recent geriatric meta-analysis, by the Geriatric Orthopedic Surgery & Rehabilitation on behalf of the NIH, National Institutes of Health, revealed that women sustaining a hip fracture had a 5-fold increase and men almost an 8-fold increase in relative likelihood of death within the first 3 months, after a hip fracture.

Most Common Reasons Seniors Fall

- Vision may decrease which can lead to falls due to not seeing clearly
- Muscle loss, hips and legs can become weaker making it harder to walk
- Poor posture or and spinal degeneration making it harder to stand erect.
- Ability to lift feet decreases with age and can stumble easily.
- It takes longer to react when something is in the way causing falls.
- Many medications interact causing dizziness or decrease balance.
- Low blood pressure can lead to light headedness and cause falls.

Add alcohol to a senior and you have an accident waiting to happen. These are a few reasons why it is most important for seniors to avoid alcohol or only consume half of a regular sized drink. Also that is why doing mind body agility exercises and beginning a balance program for seniors which incorporates strength training, endurance training and balance training is essential in maintaining and promoting good balance and maintaining good elderly health.

Baby Boomer Alcohol Epidemic

Baby Boomers are the second largest generational sector of the American population and these 75 million boomers may be reluctant to seek help for mental health issues and instead self-medicate with alcohol, which, in turn, could make them equally unlikely to get the help they would need for an alcohol dependency. There are several other key factors in play that have also contributed to the overwhelming lack of attention that has been paid to this swiftly growing problem. Many seniors who are struggling with alcohol abuse may go unnoticed due to the symptoms of alcoholism being so similar to medical and behavioral issues common among seniors, such as:

- Problems with balance and coordination
- Dementia and memory problems
- Depression
- Adult onset diseases, such as high blood pressure, diabetes, ect.
- Bad medication reactions mixing alcohol with prescriptions

Another issue is the lack of adequate screening by physicians, which can be due to either a lack of training or something far worse: a bias that alcoholism and other substance abuse disorders are “not worth the effort” of treating in seniors. In fact, this surprisingly pervasive bias is part of why there is only very limited data on how best to treat older adults struggling with alcohol dependency. Older people dealing with alcoholism often simply does not inspire the same sense of urgency that these problems do when present in younger people and is often seen as a “waste” of resources.

Chapter 9

Discouragement Despair Hopelessness

Alcoholism is a disease of despair. Discouragement is the opposite of encouragement and I believe everyone goes through periods of discouragement, so you are certainly not alone if you've been betrayed by others. We are told that God is not going to ever leave us and he will never forsake us as some people will. My mom once said, if you don't have hope you don't have anything. As long as you have hope and faith you can work to make things better. In the bible, David tells Solomon to be strong and courageous and don't be afraid or fear because God is not going anywhere. God is always there for us. The day may come when our own family members may betray us, as Jesus said, it will get so bad near the end that "Brother will deliver brother over to death, and the father his child, and children will rise against parents and have them put to death and you will be hated by all for my name's sake. But the one who endures to the end will be saved" (Matthew 10:21-22). The same applies to you and your life of sobriety no matter how hard it gets, hang in there have faith and perseverance and with God's help, self-work, abstinence and determination, you can overcome alcohol.

Self- Medicating With Alcohol

Alcohol has a numbing effect. Alcohol was used for a millenial as a pain medicine and antiseptic. Back in the days of the old west, a cowboy would take a swig of whiskey and dig a bullet out with a knife then sear the wound with a red-hot fire poker. Thank god, those barbaric days are over. Thankfully, we have many over the counter pain medication options that are non-addicting. Pain is the worst sensation of the human condition. Pain can be hard to treat because each type of pain responds to a different type of care. There can be a dull pain, throbbing pain, burning pain, stabbing pain, intermittent pain and constant pain. Pain comes in many forms and in those terrible moments, it can be really difficult to find a healthy way to deal with it. Self-medicating with alcohol for the pain becomes a familiar catch-all whether it's helping anything in the bigger picture or not.

The best natural options for pain are:

1) CBD Topical Pain Cream (see back of book for references)
2) Physical Therapy/ Therapeutic Massage
3) Exercise - mild swimming, walking, cycling

4) Hot Tub / Whirlpool (contrast therapy) hot/cold
5) Therapeutic Modalities (ultrasound, microcurrent, low level laser)
6) Mind Body Medicine (meditation/medical hypnosis/ chi gong yoga)
7) Passive Stretching
8) Vibration Massage Tapotement or fast gentle karate chopping
9) Over the counter pain meds
10) Non-Narcotic Prescription Drugs
11) Not Street Drugs That Mimic Narcotics
12) Acute Sprain Injuries (R.I.C.E. rest, ice, compression & elevation)
13) Mild-Hyperbaric Oxygen Chamber
14) Topical Rubbing Alcohol- Hydrogen Peroxide Wound Care
15) Take a sabbatical from getting intoxicated with alcoholic beverages

In fact, the risks of self medicating with alcohol, is a dangerous habit, and the risks are much greater than the short-lived relief it can offer. The more someone turns to drinking for comfort and for pain maintenance, the greater the chances of developing a dependance or an addiction.

Dual Diagnosis

Many alcoholics have a dual diagnosis, that means two or more co-existing disease states that magnifies or compounds the other. Mental health, physical health and emotional health all deteriorate when chronic alcohol abuse is an issue. When people start to have health problems, alcohol can worsen health into a snowball effect of linked health problems. The first diagnosis may be alcoholism, or alcohol use disorder, the secondary diagnosis may be bipolar affective, and additionally there may be hypertension or high blood pressure. Many overachievers that have an alcohol problem, also have an underlying psychological disorder, such as obsessive compulsive disorder OCD and they choose to drink as a form of self-medicating to try to cope with life and other people's perceived, irritating imperfections. OCD is a person who overly obsessed and has a compulsion to make things perfect. Other alcohol abusers have a dual addictions of drugs, gambling or workaholism. In these cases, their compulsion to work is similar to their addictive compulsive behavior concerning alcohol. Workaholics use work as an escape from the other regions of their life or use it to validate themselves. Success in the workplace gives them a sense of control and a sense of importance that they seek obsessively. This obsessive behavior isolates workaholics from their family and causes extreme fatigue and stress, which creates the potential of self-medication with substances.

Alcohol Waste Your Time

Waiting, Self-Medicating, Depression, Hopelessness and Impatience

Many people are depressed. Depression can mask as many other symptoms. When a person feels their life is cumbersome, or if a person feels stuck in an unhappy situation, life, relationships, job, marriage. Those with poor coping skills, may turn to alcohol as a quick fix to feel better, this is another form of self medication. If you feel let down or disappointed in life make changes to improve your situation and seek counseling. Depression may progress into clinical depression which requires professional help to pull yourself out of the depression. One day, I did some self-reflection I had been keeping myself so busy, and what seemed like a few years, was actually 10 years has flown by. Alcohol causes you to be too patient when waiting for something. I was using it to deal with the frustration of waiting for things to happen, in my life.

- Waiting and I was frustrated
- Waiting and using wine as a crutch to cope
- Waiting on others instead of doing my own thing
- Waiting to see if people would keep their word
- Waiting and it was killing me inside
- Waiting on a deal that fell through
- Waiting for a friend to keep a promise
- Waiting on a soul mate to come into my life
- Waiting for my friend to snap out of being a b_____
- Waiting on a celebrity to follow through on our deal
- Waiting on my finances to get better

Alcohol is the impatient waiter's drug of choice. Feeling let down or disappointed is a trigger for every drinker. Alcohol is a depressant that slows you down. It temporarily numbs everything but in alcohol dependence you will end of going through half your life numb and when you get sober, you will have tremors and shake with emotions that alcohol suppressed for the length of time you were a drinker. In hindsight, I have always been a person to jump in and get shit done. I am patient to a point but I don't like waiting too long on others, it causes me anxiety. I start to lose respect for others when they make plans or promises they do not keep or if they procrastinate, too long. Through this process of waiting on these people to follow through. I made a decision to quit waiting. Now, I do more things, myself or I move on quickly when people stall on agreements they have made with me. I allow others a short reasonable amount of time to follow through but not to the point to frustrate me by wasting too much of my time. I am patient to a certain extent but not beyond what is reasonable. If you snooze you loose.

Time is your Most Valuable Asset You Can't Buy Time, It is Priceless ...and once you waste it you can't get it back

Surround yourself with equally energetically paced individuals, who aren't in the habit of wasting time and stop slowing yourself down to fit in with a circle you don't fit into. Get off the alcohol check back into your life, be present, do not drink alcohol so you can be passive, do not drink to prevent yourself from getting fed up with other people's actions, cut the dead wood out of your life, face your problems head on and do not let others pull you off my own path in life or self-medicate at the point your struggles become too difficult. Seek professional advice instead of trying to self medicate and don't knock yourself out trying to accommodate other people's timelines, agendas and schedules.

Accepting Responsibility

In the aftermath, deals will come and go and I am left with myself to deal with it. I had to find my true inner self that I lost with alcohol use. There is always that one excuse. I got in the wrong personal relationships with lower energy people that couldn't keep up with my high energy and used wine to bring my energy down to their level. I was disappointed when people failed to follow through on promises they made to me and my daughter, that greatly affected her career. I was the single mom and working as the dad, too. I had many responsibilities and obligations. I have a strong integrity for myself and others. I was having some tough times with family relationships, my mother was aging and I allowed myself to self-medicating with the wine instead of taking time out to face problems head on. I viewed my wine drinking as a healthier option over following the mainstream medical approach of taking anti-depressant drugs, which were the typical treatment of the times for my symptoms. Although alcohol is quick and easy access it is not the only available option in hard times. It is a choice, no one makes you drink. You buy it. You open it.

YOU open your mouth, YOU pour it in and YOU swallow it

YOU can quit. Only you can make the choice to quit, your own drinking habit. If you feel you can't quit or if you feel you can't do it on your own, pick up the phone. There are many help hotlines with counselors that can talk you through difficult times and direct you to better treatment options.

Self-medicating with alcohol for pain can have devastating and even more painful consequences. Alcohol abuse can lead to serious risks for the body, and risks for the mind and emotions. When self-medicating becomes a pattern, professional treatment is critical to initiate recovery for substance use disorders, any co-occurring disorder, and, of course, the hidden and original sources of pain.

Alcohol is tricky to self-medicate with. At first, with just one drink, a night-cap, you get a quick relaxing effect that wears off quickly and back on with life the next day. Unlike sedative sleeping pills that make you feel groggy the next day and initially alcohol appears to pose less of a risk than the standard of care anxiety medications. Alcohol slowly depletes serotonin, the feel good hormone, in your system and eventually overtime you notice the depressant effect, usually, by then you feel depressed between drinking times. Additionally, you may notice that you feel tired and have a loss of motivation.

Mixing Alcohol With other Medications

Some of the typical anti-anxiety medication in one molecule different than cocaine and some attention enhancing medications are only one molecule short of being a methamphetamine. It is common for patients to get hooked on their medications and when they can no longer acquire the medications via prescription they resort to street drugs such as crystal meth, then you have real problems not only with addiction but legal problems as well. When a person mixes alcohol with any other mind or mood altering medication combination is disastrous and potentially deadly. It is the norm for the majority of gynecologist to recommend and prescribe antidepressants to women who suffer from premenstrual and menopausal symptoms to treat stress and anxiety, however, these medications often cause more harm than good, they create a dependency and are just masking the symptoms or emotions that are usually easily improved with proper diet, exercise, lifestyle changes and psychological counseling. Many of these medications are also not only addictive but potentially destructive or deadly as some of the side effects, actually, include suicide. Mixing any of these alcohol can be deadly.

Alcoholism is Progressive

A serving of wine is 4-6 ounces. When we first start drinking, a drink makes us feel better for a period of time, then after a while we become desensitized to the effect and end up drinking more than what is considered a single serving. In other words, alcoholism is progressive, before you realize it you graduate up to two 6 ounce glasses and then when we become tolerant of that dose before you know it you are drinking a 12 oz glass and calling it a serving, no that is 3 glasses of wine.

Signs Of Building Tolerance

- Frequently, drinking beyond feeling buzzed
- Drinking more than the daily maximum, regularly
- Instead of 1 or 2 drinks you have 3 or more, regularly
- You use to drink a 3 ounce glass an now you drink a 10 ounce glass
- you drink more than most because you have built a tolerance

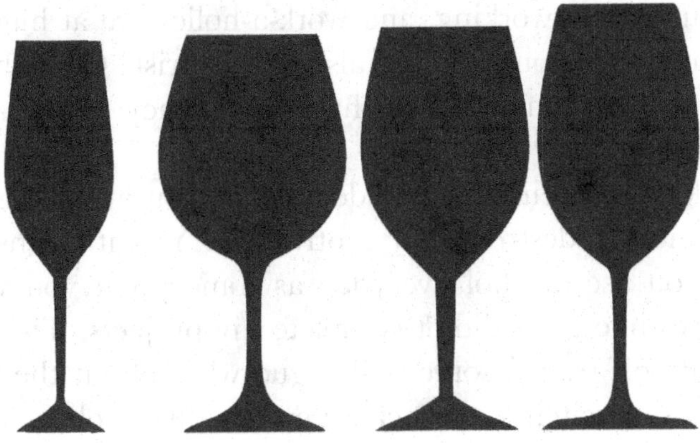

ThenNow

In every drinker's life there will come a time that you will realize your drinking more now than you used to and that you consume more than a usual amount. For some it may be instead of a glass or two of wine, you may build a tolerance to drink ½ bottle a night to get the affect, at that point you have become alcohol dependant and have developed a moderate drinking habit. At that point, it is hard to quit, cold-turkey but if you dont quit you may eventually become an alcoholic, it's that simple. The good news is, it is not true that once an alcoholic, always an alcoholic. Yes, you can recover and live a happy, comfortable life without alcohol.

Alcohol Is Flammable Play With Fire You Get Burned...

Cocaine blocks the reuptake of a few neurotransmitters, Alcohol blocks the reuptake of neurotransmitters. Alcohol is toxic, its flammable and it is more addictive than cocaine. When you quit drinking alcohol, withdrawal happens until the neurotransmitters rebalance in the brain. To put this into perspective, cocaine only blocks 11 neurotransmitters, so technically it is more difficult to stop drinking than it is to quit a cocaine habit, yet, the government classifies cocaine as a narcotic and alcohol as legal to all those who wish to use it as long as your 21 years of age. Basically, the more toxic substance is legal.

After a few years of a daily glass or 2 of wine habit, you are guaranteed one of the hardest struggles in your life when you choose to quit drinking. Alcohol leads to overeating. When we drink it also triggers our urges to snack and eat. Overeating leads to being overweight and out of shape. Alcohol is empty sugary calories that turn to fat on the body and internally around the heart and abdominal organs.

Drinking leads to over drinking and other bad habits. Alcohol is a sedative. It sedates you. Long term chronic alcohol abuse leads to a loss of physical fitness. Most people will not exercise while drinking alcohol because it is a sedative and makes you more sedentary. That is one of the hooks, especially for those of us whom are innately high energy personalities. We are the ones our mothers tell us to sit down and rest, that we are doing too much, over working, and work-a-holics are at higher risk too. Those with obsessive compulsive personalities are also more at risk. Over thinkers and chronic worriers are also at risk. Personalities that have a tendency to over-do anything are at risk to over drink once they start drinking.

Over Drinking leads to being over- sedentary. If you are a high achiever alcohol abuse has the tendency to destroy your motivation. Yes, it calms you down, but it over calms. When you use alcohol everyday as some point you will look back and say, where did all the time go. I didn't complete my projects. The alcohol eventually gets everything in life off track. Some will argue what about the highly functioning alcoholic, even in those it catches up because eventually if robs you of your health. It destroys relationships because it numbs you emotionally, It destroys your jobs because eventually it causes you to be unreliable, and have more sick days recovering from headaches and hangovers. Alcohol overuse and abuse destroys your health, your body and your mind in many ways.

How Many Drinks Are Considered Alcoholism

The definition for over-drinking varies greatly between the experts. According to NIAAA for men, low-risk alcohol consumption is considered drinking 4 or fewer standard drinks on any single day and less than 14 drinks during a week and to remain low-risk, both the daily and weekly guidelines must not be exceeded. Women who consume 8 or more drinks per week are considered excessive drinkers. And for men, excess is defined as 15 or more drinks a week. However, Dr. Kari Poikolainen, who used to work for the World Health Organization as an alcohol expert says drinking a bottle of wine a day isn't bad for you. He believes drinking only becomes harmful when people consume more than 13 units a day a bottle of wine contains 10 units. The WHO standard is considered Alcohol abuse according to NIH standards.

The Dietary Guidelines for Americans issued by the U.S. Department of Health and Human Services and U.S. Department of Agriculture.

Social Drinker-

- 1 drink per event for women on the weekend and up to 2 drinks on the weekend for men (does not drink during the work week)

Moderate Drinking -

- 1 drink per day for women and up to 2 drinks per day for men.

Binge Drinking-

- 4 drinks for women and 5 drinks for men within 2 hours. Basically, means getting smashed. NIAAA defines binge drinking as a pattern of drinking that brings blood alcohol concentration (BAC) levels to 0.08 g/dL. This typically occurs quickly in about 2 hours.
- 5 or more drinks for men and 4 or more drinks for women is the definition of binge drinking according to The Substance Abuse and Mental Health Services Administration (SAMHSA), which conducts the annual National Survey on Drug Use and Health (NSDUH) same time or within a couple of hours of each other on the same.

The First Sign of Alcoholism

The first signs of alcoholism by definition is that you drink more than you once did to get "relaxed" or buzzed. An alcoholic can therefore drink more than other people without getting drunk because they build a tolerance. Regular heavy drinkers usually have to drink more and more in order to have the same effect. In some cases, the amount of alcohol that needs to be consumed will be dangerously close to the amount that can cause alcohol poisoning. Tolerance develops because the liver produces more enzymes which is known as alcohol dehydrogenase. The enzyme is responsible for breaking down and metabolizing alcohol. Alcohol is dehydrating to your entire body and the fermentation basically pickles your liver.

Drinking alcohol pickles your organs, (juicy hydrated cucumber vrs. dried up pickle)

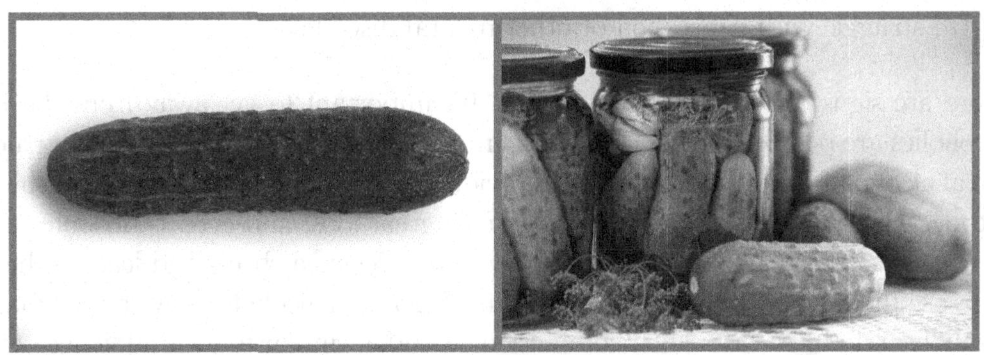

Why is getting drunk referred to as "Pickled"?
Alcohol Pickles Your Liver and Brain.

Alcohol Gene

Scientists use to believe that the presence of tetrahydroisoquinolines, alkaloid interacting proteins, could be used to determine whether someone is an alcoholic or a social drinker. However, as of yet, there has not been narrowed down to a single gene responsible for alcoholism and some experts insist there isn't one.

Some people seem to have a metabolism that processes alcohol more efficiently than the general population but it is not due to an alcohol gene. Some people seem to have a more addictive prone personality type. Many factors influence alcohol processing speed, and no two people metabolize alcohol at the exact same pace. However, alcohol processing is remarkably consistent for most individuals. As a general rule, most individuals metabolise one standard sized alcoholic drink per hour be it one beer, one glass of wine, or one shot of hard liquor, regardless of type.

Functional Alcoholism- Is a real subtype of alcohol use disorder. The National Institute on Alcohol Abuse and Alcoholism, part of the National Institutes of Health, identified five distinct "subtypes" of alcohol abusers. This dispels the notion of the "typical alcoholic".

- 19.5% of American alcoholics falls into the "functional" subtype – almost 1 out of every 5.
- Because the NIAAA estimates that there are approximately 17 million US adults with an AUD, that means there are over 3.3 million functional alcoholics in this country.
- Functional alcoholics tend to be/have:
  - Middle-aged
  - Well-educated
  - A good job
  - A stable home and family life
- 1/3 of functional alcoholics have a multi-generational family history of alcohol abuse
- 1/4 struggle with depression or other mental disorder

There are signs of functional Alcoholism. It's important to get away from the notion that alcoholics are people of low income and limited education. This simply is not true, and functional alcoholism proves it. These are individuals whose lives appear to be just fine from the outside. They may have a lot of friends, have great jobs, and even contribute in some positive ways to society but eventually, the negative affects catch up and lead to the same problems as other drinkers. Many over-achieving functional alcoholics have a dual diagnosis of workaholism. In these cases, their compulsion to work is similar to their addictive behavior to drink alcohol. Workaholics use work as an escape from problem areas of their life. Many have OCD dual diagnosis. An inflated ego and super star success in the workplace gives them a sense of power, control and a sense of exaggerated importance that they seek obsessively. This obsessive behavior isolates workaholics from their family and causes extreme fatigue and stress, which creates the potential of self-medication with alcohol and other substances.

Entertainers Alcohol Use

It takes a lot of hard work to get to the top in Hollywood and some of the top professionals in Hollywood are functional alcoholics. Money can act as a blessing or a curse. In the case of the functional alcoholic, there is a constant flow of disposable income, an addict may pay their way out of going through the horrors of withdrawal. Wealthy addicts often hire extremely skilled lawyers to rescue them from jail time or to cover up a bad legal record. If you think about all of the celebrities who have died in the past few years, or who have legal problems is is usually tied to alcohol and substance abuse issues. If they are forced to go to rehab some of the facilities are more like an expensive spa retreat and those facilities cannot treat the plethora of complexities of the functional alcoholic.

Alcohol Metabolising Enzymes - Low to Heavy Use:

Heavy alcohol use as binge drinking on 5 or more days in the past month. NIAAA's Definition of Drinking at Low Risk for Developing Alcohol Use Disorder (AUD):

1. Alcohol dehydrogenase converts alcohol into energy.
2. Cytochrome P450 2E1 is very active in the livers of chronic, heavy drinkers. This enzyme actually drains the body of energy in order to break down alcohol.
3. A third enzyme, catalase, which is present in cells throughout the body, also metabolizes a small amount of alcohol.

SPEED OF ALCOHOL METABOLISM BLOOD ALCOHOL CONTENT (BAC)

According to University of Notre Dame, time is the only factor to lower one's Blood Alcohol Content. Coffee, cold showers are all myths.

Blood/Breath Alcohol Concentration (BAC) is the amount of alcohol in the bloodstream or on one's breath. BAC is expressed as the weight of ethanol, in grams, in 100 milliliters of blood, or 210 liters of breath. BAC can be measured by breath, blood, or urine tests.

The number of drinks consumed is a very poor measure of intoxication largely because of variation in physiology and individual alcohol tolerance.

Variations exists with respect to:

- Body weight
- Gender
- Body fat percentage, even between genders

Neither blood alcohol content (BAC), nor the number of drinks consumed are necessarily accurate indicators of the level of impairment. Tolerance to alcohol also varies from one person to another, and can be affected by such factors as genetics, adaptation to chronic alcohol use, and synergistic effects of drugs. Basically, there is no safe level of drinking and driving. For example, if a drinker goes to bed at 2:00 a.m. with a BAC of .20 when they wake up at 9:00 a.m. their BAC is .095 and they're still legally intoxicated and if they drive to class and get pulled over for rolling through a stop sign they will get a DUI. It takes up to 24 hours to metabolise alcohol at 3:00 p.m. the next day, you could still have a BAC of .005 and technically, still intoxicated the next day. The following chart illustrates the effects of various blood alcohol on the physical body and the physiological impairment caused per BAC level.

Stage	BAC % Level	Feeling	Symptoms
1	.01-.04	Relaxed	Slight muscle relaxation and mood elevation
2	.05-.07	Excited/ Euphoric	Tipsy, Slurred Speech, Clumsy, Dishevelled. Slowed reaction time.
3	.08-.15	Excited/ Confused	Laughing and crying, mood swings, happy, angry, sad
4	.16-.20	Conflicted	Major impairment of mental and physical, double vision.
5	.21-.30	Stupor	Loss of Motor Control, No Control Of Mind or Body
6	.31-.40	Black-Out Coma or Death	Unconsciousness, No Reflexes, Physically Immobile Coma, Near Death
7	.41 % +	DEATH	Deep Coma & Death Respiration and Organ Failure
	QUIT	OR	DIE

Our Family's Tragic Battle With Alcoholism

In the spring of 2017, my daughter and I both had gone through two devastating personal relationship losses, the deaths of her father and my mother. I was grief stricken for my daughter, as she had a double whammy of grief, her father and her grandmother had both died only a couple months apart. Her father was the nicest person you ever met, when he was sober but when he drank to the point of blacking out, he was whole other personality. His funeral was packed, he had no shortage of friends. However, having many drinking buddies only reinforces an alcoholics tendency to drink. Alcohol can cause a tendency for the drinker to take their stress and anger out on those closest to them. He had struggled with severe alcoholism since his early 30's and we survived a living hell by divorcing out of the emotionally abusive codependent relationship that was sometimes more than just emotionally abusive. Alcohol numbs your emotions and feelings, there is no way that you can completely love and feel correctly while using alcohol. When a person, on alcohol, is not able to love and feel completely it's impossible to show their true feelings and emotions or be 100% loving and committed in an intimate relationship when you are having an affair with a bottle of alcohol.

To be in love with an alcoholic is like being in love with someone who is having an extra marital affair, except it's not an affair with another person, they have an affair with the contents of a bottle that they are in love with, it's a substance that they are addicted to the effects. You can't give 100% of yourself to someone you are given 50% of your time being drunk or pursuing an addiction to alcohol. Alcohol seems to allow the drinker to detach themselves from their problems, mentally and emotionally. Alcoholics become detached from their family and themselves and everything else. An alcoholic becomes married to the contents of the bottle.

In a sense, an alcoholic is married to alcohol.

My ex's drinking behaviors continued and we all watched in horror, 25 years of his own self-destruction, he never married again, and no amount of love from his mom and daughter, nor the rehab and counseling ordered by the courts neither seemed to help him stop.

God only knows why lives sometimes end so tragically. Before Alcohol hi-jacked his life, he wanted to conquer the world. As an adult, Alcohol robbed him of everything, including his life. It is sad to watch someone become totally consumed by alcohol to the point that it creates the circumstances that landed them in a place that they lose their life. Some people have the addiction gene, god bless them.

Military & Alcohol

My dad served in the army. Military personnel are discouraged from drinking as they risk deployment at anytime and soldiers must be alert and prepared at any time to defend our country. In December 1917, during the first world war, President Woodrow Wilson signed an alcoholic beverage proclamation to establish dry zones around military camps. The Selective Service Act forbade the sale of liquor to men in uniform. These acts were to protect soldiers and the nation, needing the protection of the soldiers. The government knew, that soldiers would be more tempted to self-medicate their stress if alcohol was readily available and that Alcohol consumption can take away having the upper hand in war. Alcohol adversely affects a soldiers mental thinking, dulls needed combat strategizing and can lead to more war time deaths. Today, some drink in groups to celebrate combat victories in social settings or alone to mask trauma. According to army statistics, 85 % of the soldiers seeking outpatient substance abuse treatment did so for alcohol. Social pressures to bury emotions can encourage active military personnel members to cope with negative emotions, such as depression by silently turning inward and drinking. Alcohol dependence can easily shift into alcoholism if they continue drinking despite potentially severe consequences to their life and the lives of others, especially if one is self-medicating traumatic military flashbacks or emotions. The Army suffered 52% of the suicides from all branches, likely because of the level of stress associated with ground combat. In 2018, 325 active army personnel committed suicide. The Marines Corps' suicide rate is at a 10-year high, also. Sadly, 75 Marines ended their own lives in 2018 and its higher for veterans, the VA study shows that roughly 22 veterans a day are dying by suicide that's 1 every 65 minutes.

Alcohol The American Terrorist

Alcohol is addictive. Alcohol use can progress into alcoholism, it's not a question of will you become addicted, it is when will you become addicted. There is no safe level of regular use. Alcohol is like a foreign terrorist invading our country and destroying the lives and futures of Americans. 32 million Americans struggle with a drinking problem. 13.8 million Americans are alcoholics. Alcohol is a deadly body-snatcher that claimed the lives of 88,000 fellow Americans, last year. There is a war against Alcoholism and we are losing the battle.

Rock Bottom Or Intervention

At some point, the alcoholic hits rock bottom and family members usually make a choice to do an intervention and stop enabling the alcoholic. Many times an intervention and rehab helps the alcoholic stop drinking but more often than not, they eventually begin drinking again and it's a vicious cycle with no peace for the families affected unless, the alcoholic chooses on their own to quit drinking themselves. Don't wait until it is too late.

When An Alcoholic Hits Rock Bottom The ONLY Way Out Is To Quit or Die

Sadly, the only option left after rock bottom is to head back up and for those who don't chose to go up from rock bottom, go down in the ground dead and buried, usually, from some alcohol related situation. In our family, my ex would not quit and 25 years after our divorce, sadly, alcohol overdose .385 blood alcohol level without any medical attention was the cause of his death. I knew how much he loved me from the beginning, and for something to take over a person's mind the way it did, to change that person so far away from who they really are, I knew for sure that when I left, that he would be an alcoholic for the rest of his life, I foresaw no hope in having a healthy marriage because of alcohol and everyday he lived was a surprise. He obviously one of those rare people who had the enzyme or gene of addiction. It has been a heartbreaking ordeal for my daughter her whole life, its sad she never got to know her dad before alcohol addiction and we always planned to put him in a better rehab facility in California. One night, a couple of years after his death, I was reviewing the autopsy records, it was heartbreaking to see how horrible the final hours of his life was. Seeing those horrible death reports definitely would influence any drinker to make the decision to quit and live a life of sobriety.

Rock Bottom Skid Row

Estimates of the number of homeless people in the United States today vary considerably from a low of 250,000 to as many as 3 million. However, the numbers are growing. Homelessness is a critical problem and the homeless population is plagued with serious health problems, including the heavy use of alcohol and drugs which heighten the morbidity rate among the population. The "chronic severe" alcoholic subtype is what comes to mind when someone thinks of an "alcoholic" someone who may be homeless, drunk more often than not, and unable to function normally in society. The City of Los Angeles is skid row capital of the U.S. There are over 25,000 homeless, 76% experience alcohol, drug or mental health problems, Sadly, of the total, over 6,000 of the homeless are veterans which is an indication of the roll of post traumatic stress as a major factor of veterans self-medicating with alcohol. The Homeless Population with

Alcohol and Other Drug Problems

The results of recent research on the prevalence of alcohol and other drug problems among homeless persons are particularly clear on one point: that alcohol and other drug problems constitute the number one public health problem among this population. Studies conducted during the 1980s show that 30% of homeless people have alcohol problems and 10% had histories of other drug problems. Today's homeless population is more diverse than in the past. It includes women, children, families, adolescents, people of color, the mentally ill, and users of other drugs and skid row alcoholics. Their lives tend to be marked by multiple risk factors, including poverty and use of alcohol and drugs. Skid row is a phase after hitting rock bottom and before death.

When You Realize Alcohol Is Killing You Your Health Becomes More Valuable To You Than Any Pleasure Or Relief You Had From Alcohol

Chapter 10

Solutions To Reverse the Effects of Drinking

You can reverse the effects of drinking. Depending on the length and severity of an untreated drinking problem and the degree of damage already done, you can reverse some if not all of alcohol's effects on the brain and liver, according to the latest scientific research. The solution lies within this book by utilizing these quick, effective tips and home-care treatments to help prevent Alcohol dependence and lessen the negative effects of Alcohol use. Usually, all light drinkers and most moderate drinkers will be able to quit on their own with this self-detox plan because it offers simple and easy-to-follow methods of detoxing from alcohol on your own with minimal difficult and without the intense discomfort of detoxing cold-turkey, on your own. Statistically, over time, drinkers progress into the disease of alcoholism and 1-5% will require medical detox or they could die of DT's (delirium tremens) without medical assistance. The odds are you are one of the lucky majority of people who will be able to self-detox without medical intervention with these Safe And Effective Self-Care Tips that Help Curb Alcohol Cravings.

Quitting Is The Solution Here And Abroad

Many relatives of drinkers who are struggling with substance abuse are ashamed of the problem and will choose to ignore it rather than admit that they need help. For seniors suffering from alcohol dependence, it is vital that they get the help they need, which is why breaking down stigmas that still surround both mental illness and substance abuse to some degree is so important. Never quit encouraging your loved ones to quit drinking. We can adopt better public health and alcohol awareness campaigns like other countries. For example, the University of Sussex reported that their "Dry January" public health campaign is working to reduce alcohol abuse throughout the United Kingdom. Participants also had several other positive benefits:

- 82 % felt a sense of achievement
- 79 % saved money,
- 62 % had better sleep,
- 62 % had more energy and
- 49 % lost weight.

Staying dry for January may also help jump-start people to give up alcohol for longer. Although most people who participate in Dry January return to drinking, up to 8 percent stay dry six months later, according to Public Health England and the British Medical Journal.

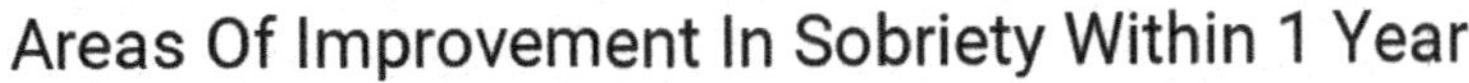

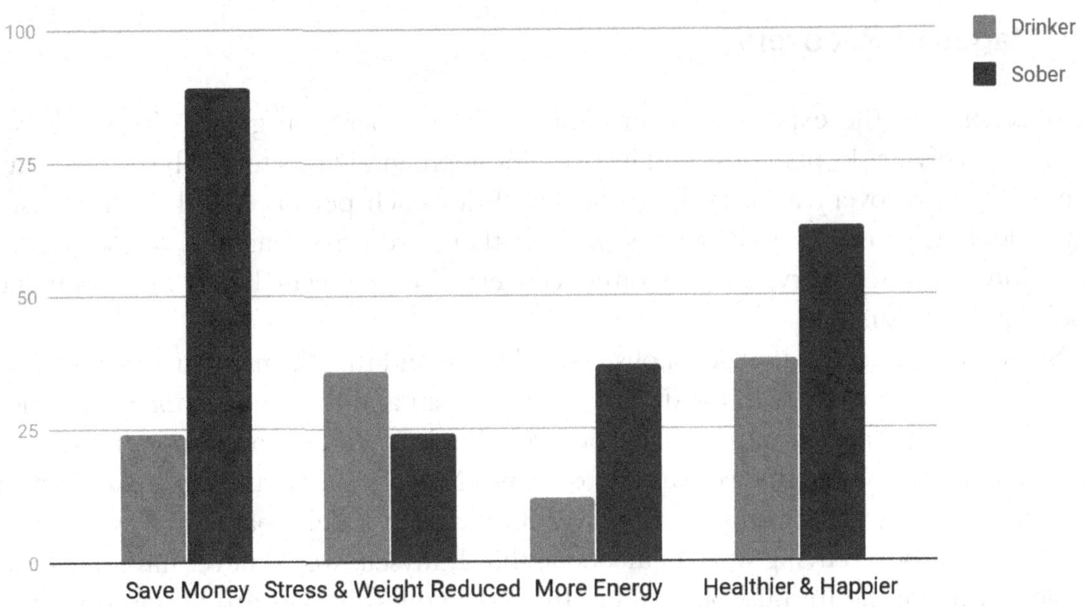

Deciding How To Quit

In a national epidemiologic survey on alcohol and related conditions, it was determined that 70% of alcohol users quit on their own or cut back to healthful levels without institutionalized treatment. 29 % needed some additional assistance in quitting, seeking one or more medical providers. However, 1% suffered severe alcohol addiction who relapsed to rock bottom. This study was the largest recorded and most comprehensive survey of drinking cessation, thus far. Other nationally recognized addiction experts have also stated, that the traditional approaches to alcohol treatment have been too narrow in their approach to correcting alcohol disorders. Another five year alcohol research project surveyed 43,000 chronic alcohol users from 2001-2005 with the most remarkable finding of the study revealing just how great of a problem alcohol abuse is amongst the majority of adult Americans. Americans are experiencing an epidemic of "alcohol-use-disorder" AUD. The AUD label qualifies as either abuse or dependence at some point during the test subjects lifetime and the study concluded that approximately 70% of the chronic drinkers in the survey reported having quit and recovered on their own. About 30% of Americans had experienced a disorder, the research showed, but about 70% of those quit drinking or cut back to safe levels of consumption without treatment within the time span of the five year study. The most widely used traditional recovery treatment model used is designed for the worst 1% of alcoholics. Hopefully, you may be like one of the 70% who quit on their own but if you are in the 1% you will likely need to continual follow a lifelong 12 step program, go through periodic institutionalized rehab programs and regular counseling for sobriety support.

Stages of Recovery

According to the experts, recovery is a process of personal growth in which each stage has its own risks of relapse and its own developmental tasks to reach the next stage. The stages of recovery are not the same length for each person, but they are a useful way of looking at recovery. Broadly speaking, there are three stages of recovery called transition, early recovery, and ongoing recovery. More recent labels are abstinence, repair, and growth.

Some experts believe that Alcoholism is a disease and that former drinkers are always classified as an alcoholic with the disease of alcoholism and that an alcoholic is an addict who is forever and always in recovery. For some that is true, there are those drinkers that fall in that category and my ex- was one of those. My ex's over drinking broke everyone in his family's heart, over and over for over 35 years on a daily basis. You would think after having survived living with an alcoholic that I, myself, would never have a drinking problem. I made the mistake of thinking that Alcoholics drank hard liquor, my ex was a whiskey and vodka drinker which I never drank. 25 years later, I made my own mistake of thinking wine, wasn't really alcohol like hard liquor, because wine was the first medicine and wine is a sacrament in the bible. Not true, being a wino is the same as being an alcoholic.

Alcohol Dependance Creeps Up On You

For years, I could not see the gradual negative affect that wine was having on me. I did not realize alcohol dependency was creeping up on me and I was slowly building up a tolerance. We teach our kids not to smoke or use illegal drugs, we teach them about not talking to strangers, to fear abductors, we don't teach them enough about why and how that substances can grab them and hijack their lives. Alcohol starts out fun then gradually the ugly addiction side of it, grabs you, hijacks your life and holds you hostage, in many ways. Wine numbed my emotions enough that I didn't feel upset that my marriage didn't work out, eased the pain of hurtful things that insensitive family members said or did to me and I used wine to numb my pain and frustrations. Alcohol seemed like it helped me feel better while it was only wasting my time, robbing me of motivation and side tracking me from facing my problems head on. Alcohol made me not care enough that I temporarily didn't feel upset about life's many struggles that we all have to deal with. I could not see, that Alcohol was mostly an obstacle that made me procrastinate and miss many opportunities. Alcohol sedates you and steals your motivation. Alcohol caused me to have poor judgement because I wasn't feeling or thinking clearly.

One day, on a trip down south, to visit my mom she said to me, I can see from your appearance, that you've been working hard out in California. I said mom, it's just the jet lag from the 3,000 mile journey home. At times that was true but at that time I viewed myself as being highly functioning wine drinker and successful in my business. My daughter was loving her life, college and her friends. I was loving my career and felt my professional life had purpose because I was helping so many people improve their health and I was working in some of the most prestigious celebrity clinics in the world. It was an exciting time. Staying busy keeps your mind off other things and personal matters. It distracted me of the fact that I had, supported my daughter as a single parent for 20 years with no support from anyone and that my ex was still in the same place drinking himself to death daily, often by the time I would get back home to visit mom I would be utterly exhausted from the intense pressure of my work schedule and the exhaustive travel.

The trip home was always a refuge for me, early on, it was a once a year opportunity to get away from my drill sergeant of a boss and later after opening my own business, it was a much needed time off to catch up with my mother away from the hustle of the big city. Unfortunately, it was a grueling 3 day car trip through the desert or a 3,000 mile red-eye flight so regardless of the method of transportation, by the time I arrived to visit my mom I was usually exhausted and would sleep the better part of the next day. Usually, I would fly home and when I flew I had so many miles racked up I would usually get bumped to an unsold 1st class seat where they served all the wine and champagne you wanted, so I took advantage on those occasions and by the time my flight would arrive, I would be a little tipsy even just from 2 glasses of wine, and of course, flight intensifies the effect. Then I would sleep in late the next day because of the 2-3 hr time zone difference between east and west coast, travel makes you look like you have a hangover when your sleeping in but actually the body needs a day to adjust to time zone differences, also.

My mom would be excited to make our family rounds and see everyone but then I would be off to a late start from the jet lag she not being an experienced at air travel misconstrued my condition as being hungover. Both conditions have similar symptoms, so it was confusing to her as she has never had flown very much and when she had, years before there were short flights. I explained to her, that I'm not hungover, and that I usually only drank a little wine to calm my nerves for flight jitters and to sleep at night, because i did not believe in taking drugs or medications for stress. Then mom reminded me, very tenderly of something. She said, Joy, I know you don't drink hard alcohol because of what you went through with your ex, but people can become a "Wino", also. I said, mom, I'm not a wino I have jet-lag, still, I had never thought about wine that way and I had never heard anyone make that distinction to me before and it hit me like a ton of bricks. Alcohol is alcohol, be it whiskey or wine, period. She was right.

Living With Anxiety And Parenting Without Drugs

I have always been a high energy person and its always been hard for the people around me to keep up with me but it was always hard for me to relax for years. Many different people from my mom, grandparents, teachers, colleagues and several significant others have always told me I do too many things at once. I have always been an amped up kind of person, naturally, without drugs. I have always been into fitness, I was a majorette, a cheerleader and a dancer. When my baby was born, I was determined to get my pregnancy weight off, so I was out jogging with the stroller from the 3rd week after my delivery, it was great she was a happy baby, always laughing, my own live, little baby tender love doll she was doing leg lifts with me at 6 months old and walking at 9 months she was smart and as she grew I realized she was more of an intellectual than me, she was reading her own nursery books by the time she was a year old. Once, upon a time, I was a single mom rushing around every morning to get my daughter off to a christian pre-school and to get myself to work on time, we were running about 15 minutes late and as I was putting my little 4 year olds clothes on her very quickly, it was too fast for her and she didn't like it, she grabbed both of my wrist and looked up at me square in the eye and said, its ok mommy, slow down and take care of me. I realized that my anxious energy was affecting my daughter negatively and had to do something about it. I don't do drugs so I was not the type to take a chill pill I've always loved exercising so I studied, took the test and became a certified fitness trainer so I could channel my energy into helping others get fit. I worked in an all women's gym and worked up to the fitness director position managing all the other female trainers. Still, at home I burned my daughter out going on too long hikes around the neighborhood lake trails, while I was at work, she was at school and taking swimming and music lessons and she loved swimming, that was her sport, she was on the swim team, and she practiced and became a champion in breast-stroke and won lots of competitions. Work and school can come between parents and children, so since she loved the swimming and the water, I bought me and my daughter jet skis so we could spend more time together in the water and get some exercise and have fun being together, eventually, she grew tired of it and would end up docking hers on the dock of a friends house on the lake while I was jumping barge waves and half killing myself, after that she got into her hobbies, acting, art and creative writing and I still needed an outlet for my nervous energy and stress. In her high school, years I found Mind Body Medicine, yoga and meditation which led me on a lifelong love of Ayurvedic and Natural Medicine.

Managing Stress and Anxiety With Mind Body Medicine

I wrote an exercise program it was the first that integrated yoga with traditional fitness, called the Mind Body Exercise Program and I contacted and teamed up with the Mind Body Center for Medicine which was owned by the president of the American Health Research Institute, Dr. Amrik Walia, former head of surgery at UAB medical school. There I trained in the Deepak Chopra Creating Health Instructors program and became a Mind Body medicine health coach. Mind Body medicine is a safe and effective way to manage many health problems without drugs or alcohol. In addition, to exercise, this was another way I learned to manage my nervous energy without wine.He took a great interest in my program and suggested and encouraged me to write a medical weight loss program and I did, it is called the Mind-Body Type Diet, and since patients were losing an average of 11 pounds in a week treatment program, without reducing their caloric intake. I wrote a self-help version of the program and the name of that book is "The Balance Diet and Lifestyle" it is available on Amazon and Barnes and noble. Even though I was surrounded by some of America's top health researchers and was working with some of the greatest scientific researchers in the world. They were my mentors. One of the most brilliant German cancer researchers in the world, once told me salt, always and wine, too! I observed many of these brilliant professors heavily over indulging with drinking and eventually, I did it, too.

Emotional Eaters & Emotional Drinkers

There are "emotional-drinkers". People who overeat are often "eating away their emotions, therefore thy are emotional eaters. For them, it's not what they are eating, it's what is eating them. Alcohol abuse is the same in many ways. It's not what your drinking it's about why you are drinking. What is drowning you, emotionally?

Alcohol is the 3rd leading lifestyle-related cause of death in the nation.

Loneliness and Alcohol

We are in an age of compulsive use of digital technology, sedentary lifestyle and hyper use of social media allowing us to post daily selfies and watch each others every move but studies show 1 out of 3 adults still feel lonely. Even though we can get many "likes" on our post, it's harder to get our friends to call us back. Researchers show that feeling lonely is rampant in America. Loneliness is not about feeling alone, it's the feeling that you don't feel important to anyone or feeling that no one really loves you, or feeling like no one understands and accepts you with unconditional love. Loneliness has negative effects on our health, too. Loneliness is as damaging to your health as smoking a half a pack of cigarettes per day. People who are lonely are more sick with symptoms and ailments and are 50% more likely to die before their time. Half of Americans say they have do not have meaningful face to face interactions with the people in their lives, every day. 54% say that they don't know one person that really knows them very well. 56% of people said the people they dont' feel deeply connected to the people they have surrounded themself with. 40% feel isolated and lonely several times per week and many try to self-medicate their loneliness with alcohol. Spend time with people that connect to you deeply so your future is not as lonely as the past. Being surrounded by people but not feeling, loved, cared for and understood is the root of loneliness. Start by loving yourself more, put down the alcohol and get in touch with your good qualities and then surround yourself with more loving people and work on strengthening the love in the relationships that you already have. Shocking truth about loneliness is it is the number one reason that people drink and use alcohol as an emotional crutch for emotional pain. In the study, generation Z was the loneliest of all generations. 54% say they don't know one person that knows them well. Don't have meaningful relationships but don't feel understood. Volunteer to spend time deepening your sense of purpose. It's not just being around people but being understood. Decreasing loneliness is an important first step to quitting drinking so it is important to get out of the house and do things start walking drinking lots of water and joining a support group so you don't feel lonely during alcohol detox. Finding your inner strength with like minded individuals, other quitters, talking it out in a support group that understands what your going through. Learning tips on how to navigate without alcohol in any and every situation gives you great strength and power to be successful in sobriety. Instead of going to the pub or happy hour, go to the gym, go walking, join a hiking club and exercise with others, it helps your mind and body start functioning normally again.

Missed Opportunities In Life

Missed opportunities are a reason that many people drink. When a person feels like they missed out on something in life, it can be depressing. Twice, in my life I was offered academic college scholarships, once from the University of Alabama, I was supposed to be a college majorette and earn a medical degree there and another missed opportunity, a scholarship to Wake Forest, which was the first college of medical genetics and genomics which I was not in a position to accept. Instead, I opted to take the Mind Body Medicine program at Harvard and it has helped me better help many others but many may feel they missed something they really wanted to do in life and it is a source of depression and often people try to drink their disappointments away instead of setting attainable goals and some become alcoholics.

My Mistake Of Coping With Wine

As I mentioned before, people have often had to tell me to sit down and rest that I do too much. I drank wine to unwind and settle down but also to stop pacing the floors in the evenings, usually only a glass or two of wine at a time a few times a week but, all the while I was in denial that it was becoming a problem. Wine was my part of method of relaxing and not taking stress or anxiety pills. I thought I had control over wine for 10 or more years, and I always managed to not exceed the limit I set for myself. Many people can effectively, eat and drink in moderation. Some always seem to go to extremes in everything they do. All human beings have the potential of healing from many things if they, have faith, and believe and truly want to get better and are willing to take the necessary steps and do the hard work through the painful recovery process many can transform their lives into one that they find a new joy of living in sobriety.

Getting Into A Quitter's Mindset

I was able to quit when I was able to take a mature and responsible look at my wine drinking. I wanted to become a woman that my mother would be more proud of, a good person who can help others and add value to the world, a good mother to my child and other children and I believe everyone needed me to be sober and helpful. I admitted that I did not want to allow my drinking to become a bigger problem and I made a decision to quit. I believe the body is self-healing and that anyone can recover from many illnesses if they will do the work required to correct the problem. This belief helped me get into a quitter's state of mind. Believe you can do it, believe you can quit.

Stress As A Factor in Alcohol Dependence

Stress is a silent killer. Many people have poor coping skills, and feel they have very few options to manage extreme stress. Many turn to alcohol to kill their stressful emotions and use alcohol as a quick fix to feel better. If you drink alcohol to get rid of stress jitters that is considered self-medicating with alcohol. I myself became stressed during my PhD thesis and upcoming graduation plus trying to deal with some personal difficulties and troubled family relationships. I had insomnia from worrying and that was another one of my excuses for self-medicating with wine. After those 10 years, during a period of high stress, I began drinking a glass of wine every night before bed for over a year. Daily use of alcohol leads to higher tolerance and after my graduation ceremony we binged out on wine. Some celebration, I felt like shit the next day! I knew it wasn't good for my health and I couldn't believe that it was happening to me. I had slowly built up a tolerance, and I never felt drunk util that graduation binge. I knew it was time to quit.

Alcohol And Self Harming Behavior

Abusing alcohol is a form of self-harming behavior just as over eating and other glutinous habits are. Mixing alcohol with pain medicine, antidepressants, antipsychotics or behavior medications is a death wish. The psychology of self-harm is a complex subject that requires professional help.

Drug Residues In Tap Water Dangerous Mix With Alcohol

America is only 5% of the world's population however Americans consume 80% of the narcotic pharmaceutical medications sold each year and unfortunately, it is showing up in our drinking water. Waste water is recycled in Researchers have found that many water filtration systems very rarely effectively filter out all drugs from tap water as the particulates are too small to be completely filtered out. There are approximately 4.25 billion prescriptions for antidepressants sold to Americans for over 210 billion annually, in the U.S. The earth has naturally recycled and reused water for millions of years. Water recycling, though, generally refers to projects that use technology to speed up these natural processes. In 2008, after surveying results from the municipalities that tested tap water for drugs, the associated press (AP) found over 50 pharmaceuticals that "could harm humans" in the water of 41 million Americans.

Research Example Of Hidden Drugs In Water:

- Southern California: a portion of drinking water that supplies 18.5 million people contained traces of anti-epileptic and anti-anxiety drugs.

This is only one example and most cities don't test their water for pharmaceutical residues. The actual number of people who are exposed is much higher now than these studies indicate. Even if you drink bottled water, it is likely that you are getting some drug residues in tap water, ice, cooking or making water based pictures of liquids such as tea at home and in restaurants. Therefore, mixed cocktails may also contain trace amounts of other drugs inadvertently via ice and some mixers. Many of these drugs are labeled "do not take or mix with alcohol. Therefore, even if you are not taking a prescription when drinking alcohol, you may be ingesting them accidentally through tap water. This is important to be aware of because many medications are dangerous when mixed with alcohol.

Alcohol With Prescription Medication Dangers

Mixing alcohol and medicines puts you at risk for dangerous reactions. Alcohol and medicines can interact harmfully even if they are not taken at the same time. Hundreds of medications interact with alcohol, leading to increased risk of illness, injury and in some cases death. Protect yourself by avoiding alcohol while you are taking a prescription medication and don't know its effect. When you do something that is bad for your health it always catches up with you. For example, I never take prescription pain pills because from the beginning of my life every time an M.D. ever prescribed them to me, they affected me in a horrible way. I remember only a few times in life where I was forced to take them. Once when I was a teenager and had a fractured skull from a majorette routine, gone wrong and got hit in the face with a high flying batton, that landed me in hospital with a facial hematoma and cracked skull, the MD gave me darvocet to take after release, it made me bedridden, so I didn't take them after the first day. Next time was while in hospital after the birth of my daughter and the last time I had some dental work done and was taking antibiotics and some prescription ibuprofen for the pain and swelling as a result of my dental surgery. Also, the night before, not thinking, I had drank a couple of glasses of wine and everyone knows your not suppose to drink when your on most prescription medications. I woke up one day just like every other morning, nothing unusual. It was a beautiful sunny California morning, and there I was, just finished my morning coffee and BAM! The pain hit me, like a bolt of lightning struck through my chest and the pain was so intense and piercing, it felt like I had been shot through the heart or like an arrow went straight through my heart and out my back, I felt faint, like I was blacking out, I felt the blood leave my face and I couldn't move paralyzed with pain. I couldn't even breathe. I was having a bad reaction with the antibiotic and pain med, and I thought I was having a heart attack.

WARNING: Do Not Drink Alcoholic Beverages While Taking This Medication. Mixing Medication With Alcohol May Result In Adverse Reactions Including Death.

I broke out in a cold sweat. Luckily, a friend of mine was there to help at that moment. He wanted to call 911 but I already had realized what I had done, taken my dental surgery prescription medications with alcohol the night before. I convinced my friend, that it was too late to have my stomach pumped and I knew the exact emergency medical antidote and steps to take care of my own situation but needed help mixing the antidote together to manage my urgent health crisis. I started drinking distilled water, the molecular structure of the water attaches to anything in excess and helps pull it out of the body along with my emergency remedy to flush and rapid detox my system, basically, activated charcoal and a heparin like herb with a high dose of magnesium and hawthorne and a heart compound remedy with a dozen cardiovascular ingredients poured into the distilled water for me to drink my rescue remedy, after I drank it and within 20 minutes the attack subsided but it was days before I felt anywhere back to normal again.

If my friend had not been there I'm sure I would not have been able to put together the remedy to pull myself out of the health crisis and I may have even had a heart attack. Regardless, I knew the self-medicating with wine and the stress from a strained personal relationship was a factor, but the biggest reason for me having an anxiety attack, in the first place was being under extreme stress and mixing dental prescriptions with wine, a huge no-no. Regardless, I knew I had made a stupid mistake, that many people make. Luckily for me it was only adverse reaction compounded by acute stress instead of a heart attack. I blamed the troubled family relationship but I made the wrong decision and had drank wine with antibiotics and ibuprofen.

I wasn't getting drunk but that doesnt matter with chronic alcohol consumption, as even the smallest amount of alcohol destroys your health and if compounded by stress hormones it has an accumulative effect on your heart. I remembered that my mom told me my grandmother died at 33 years old of a heart condition.

Alcohol Cannot Be Mixed With Medication, It Can Kill You.

Even the most common over the counter medications can have a random bad interaction or a rare interaction that can kill you. I thought she had rheumatic fever and that caused her weak heart, but apparently it runs in my family. I began to take a serious interest in my own heart health.

Hidden Toxins And Congeners In Alcohol

Most alcoholic beverages contain toxic additives and residues known as congeners. They are created during the fermentation process. Congeners are some of the strongest compounds known to man. They contribute to the distinct flavors of various alcoholic beverages. They interact with your body chemistry and they can be detected in your bloodstream hours after consumption. Ethanol is a chemical that is made during the distillation and fermentation process which also creates other toxic congeners chemicals such as:

- Congeners-worse in dark liquors rather than light colored ones.
- Furfuryl: Stops yeast from metabolizing.
- Methanol: Breaks down in formaldehyde & formic acid
- Tannins: antioxidants in wine.
- Fossil oil: by product of distillation process of alcoholic spirits.
- Acetaldehyde: A toxic cancer causing agent from the breakdown of ethanol.

Acetaldehyde Cancer Risk

Overtime, alcohol destroys your health, as all of the toxins and poisons accumulate in your body and are stored in fat by the buildup of acetaldehyde. Although it is not greatly recognized in the United States, according to the World Health Organization, Acetaldehyde is now classified by its International Agency for Research on Cancer as a carcinogen for humans. Acetaldehyde is a group-one cancer-causing agent that occurs by the metabolism of alcoholic beverages when there is not enough metabolic compounds to break it down and eliminate it from the body. It is one of the main reasons we gain weight around the waist from drinking, also. If bacterial microbes in your body cannot break down the acetaldehyde consumed in alcoholic beverages, it can lead to oral cancer, throat cancer, and similar alimentary tract cancers. The accumulation of acetaldehyde levels becomes a cancer risk as it has the ability to cause cancer at levels above 100 micromolar. Most all alcoholic beverages are over 100 micromolar of acetaldehyde.

One known weapon we have against acetaldehyde is the amino acid L-Cysteine, as it helps break down and neutralize acetaldehyde. Also, brushing and flossing your teeth and drinking water dilutes and decreases the micromolar levels of acetaldehyde. In the following chart, 20 = 200 micromolar and 100 = 1000 micromolar.

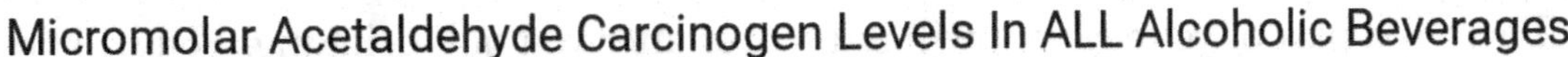

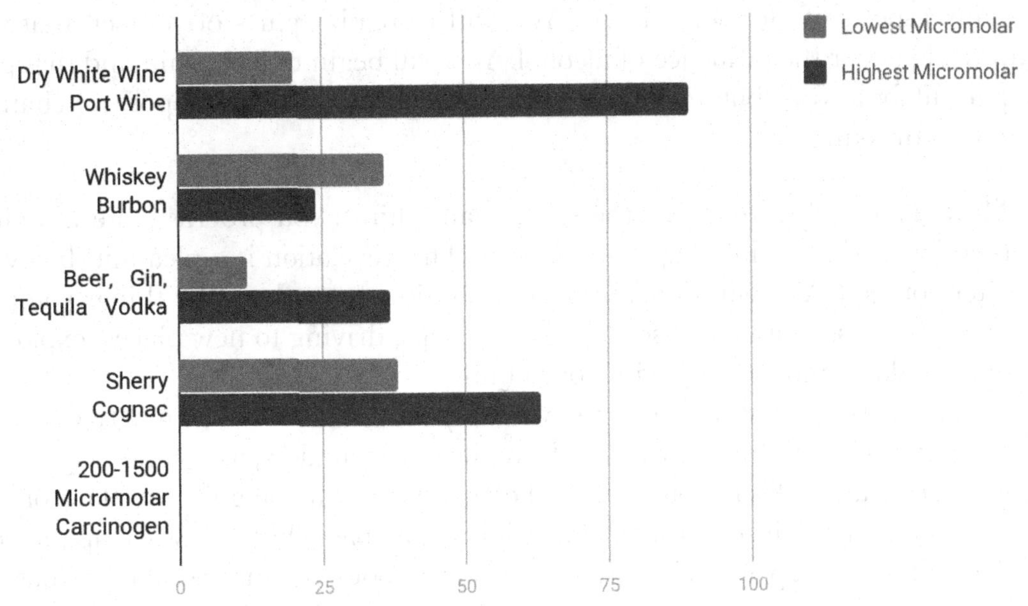

Alcohol Break Up

Just like a bad romance, at some point you know you have to end it. I decided to break-up with alcohol and just like a bad love-affair, sometimes it's a love-hate relationship. I cut back on the wine to ½ glass every other night through the week and started a heart health treatment plan. After returning from the annual medical conference and my PhD graduation trip. I had another milder angina episode, in my sleep I went into atrial fibrillation again but this time I took the remedy and the angina subsided but I knew I had to make that choice to clean up everything that was stressful in my life or progress toward a heart attack. My stress was mostly, from the heartaches that I had been carrying around. I had to learn to let stress go and to forgive and forget. I had to cut some people out of my life that were not so good for me. That is also when I decided either I have to quit drinking or die. I chose to quit ruminating over the relationship disappointments and start working on bettering my health and my life. I needed time to focus on fixing me and healing my broken heart.

Once You Realize The Risk Outweigh Fake Benefits, You May Choose To Quit

How Life Improves After You Quit

There is a part of yourself you will rediscover after you quit drinking. You will begin to see many aspects of life more clearly. You will recognize parts of yourself that was dormant while under the influence of alcohol. You will begin to feel again and that part can be painful for a while but it gets better. Here are a few examples of positive changes after you quit drinking.

- More Time- when drinking there are many things you procrastinate in doing, therefore, drinking takes up a lot of time. This revelation is a pleasant discovery after you quit. You will find you have spare time to work on the things you may have put off such as, exercise, sight-seeing trips, driving to new places, exploring life and doing more things with your family.
- Less Anxiety- at first during detox you may have a little more anxiety but soon. once through withdrawal, you will have much less anxiety, as you no longer have to worry if alcohol is in your system the next day when you go out in the world to do more things. The old drinker's worries, feeling bad when you wake up the next day will soon disappear. If you're a naturally anxious you may still be anxious but in general the mood swings will be much better than the highs and lows of getting off alcohol which is a depressant.
- Sleep Better- passing out after drinking is not equivalent to getting a good night's rest in fact, our body works hard trying to process and get rid of the alcohol so it never gets the chance to actually recuperate. In sobriety, sleep patterns will improve. After your quit, you will rest better and feel refreshed in the morning.
- Improved Mental Health and Brain Function- All the agitation alcohol can cause begins to improve and you feel happier because after all, alcohol is a depressant. Also, the foggy headed feeling from drinking too much the previous night, is gone forever. You are most likely to wake up feeling clear headed and ready to take on the world and any challenge you may face.
- Younger Looking Skin- Alcohol is dehydrating and dries your skin out, once you quit, your kidneys aren't under duress to the extent they were when you drank, so the water you drink will hydrate your cells and tissues better and your skin will show it. You will lose that dull look and start to glow again.
- No More Worry and Guilt -No more hiding your empty bottles because you're embarrassed at how much you drink. No more feeling embarrassed that the restaurant ask if you want a glass of wine at 11 am or your local store salesperson knows you by your alcohol purchases. No longer worry if you have waited long enough to drive. The list goes on.

Chapter 11

How To Quit Drinking

Many people with a drinking problem are not comfortable going to common support group meetings. Personal safety is important when choosing a support group as many violent criminals are mandated to go to recovery support groups which may not be the best support for some individuals. Not everyone can afford professional help at an expensive in patient rehab clinic. But there are many outpatient options and alternative ways of giving up alcohol. It is possible for some individuals to quit drinking alcohol, quietly, in your own home. Some simple strategies can help a recovering alcoholic beat the bottle without spending a lot of money. However, it is wise to get a medical checkup first.

When a person quits cold turkey, the first 72 hours of abstinence from alcohol are the toughest. This is the most difficult part of recovery as the body tries to reestablish a biochemical balance. This period of acute withdrawal can be unpleasant and for some it may be dangerous. Some people, especially heavy drinkers and people who have been drinking for a long time, may require professional help to get through this phase of rehab.

It is not unusual to feel anxious, restless, excited, or shaky when quitting. For severe symptoms, such as high blood pressure, tremors, seizures, and signs suggestive of delirium tremens, it is imperative to seek medical attention. To safely detox at home, it is a good idea to enlist the support of family and friends and consider taking some time off from work. Seizures are usually brief, generalized, tonic-clonic in nature, and without an aura. Status epilepticus may occur in 3% of alcohol withdrawal. It is also important at this time to focus on a balanced healthy diet and stay well hydrated.

Sick & Tired of Feeling Sick & Tired

Airplane Flight Going Down On Alcohol Dependance

When a plane is going down, the rule is grab the oxygen mask for yourself before you help others. It was time to help myself. I took a selfie-vakay, time away, as a physician, to heal myself. As a healthcare provider, my rock bottom, was a sign that my health was in jeopardy and that my stress was out of control more than it had ever been in my life. I had lost my mom, my daughter lost her dad, I had just finished up the busiest summer season at work and I had some seriously stressful personal situations. The pressure I had endured over the last few months was too much at once. I had not even began to process any of the recent traumatic events, emotionally. Fall was ending and my work was slowing down for the slow winter season. I decided to make some positive healthy lifestyle changes starting by eliminating environmental stress factors. I cleaned out my house and my office and did a makeover of environment to create my own healing space. I redecorated with purification colors, white and gold. I read the golden book, prayed and meditated, daily. I was beginning to detoxing my body from alcohol. I had a quit-drinking wine action plan in place and it started by cleaning up my environmental triggers.

The First Step To Recovery

The first step, is to have a desire to quit and admit there is a problem. The second step is to educate yourself and face denial issues. Third step is to face the fact that you have been over-drinking, admit that you have been in denial and get your head wrapped around the idea of saving your own life because alcohol has become a threatening problem in your life before you develop the deadly disease of alcoholism. The next step is making the commitment to make a lifestyle change and quit over drinking, educate yourself so you understand why alcohol became a crutch and a problem in your life. Educate yourself on the dangers, the pro's and con's. Know what to expect as you go through detox and devise a strategy on how to prevent relapse and then is the final and hardest part is completing detox and the prevention of relapse. Knowing what to expect during detox will help you to prepare, knowing what to expect through sober living stage of recovery and knowing how to protect yourself from triggers that risk a relapse and how to live a successful life of sobriety.

Euphoria Is A State Of Joy, Dysphoria Is The Opposite

Dysphoria is a state of unease, anxiety, and misery. The NIH states that one of the side effects of alcohol detoxification is Dysphoria, a state of mental discomfort or suffering. When you detox from alcohol, you may feel dysphoria and you may feel depressed and dysphoric, for a short time until your brain begins to produce endorphins and other feel good neurotransmitters and your body resumes a more balanced hormone balance. I felt dysphoria, after about the fourth week after I quit drinking, I would have random sudden burst of feeling like I wanted to cry. The dysphoria would pass almost as quickly as the feeling came. You may feel dysphoria, but when it's all over, it will be worth it. Research on the internet before and after photos of people who quit alcohol, you will look and feel so much better after detox.

Acute Withdrawal Syndrome (AWS) & Post Acute Withdrawal Symptoms (PAWS)

Acute withdrawal (AWS) will usually occur in the first week and some of the common symptoms are:

- Agitation
- Anxiety
- Cold Sweats
- Depression
- Insomnia
- Malice/Fever
- Fatigue/Tiredness
- Sadness
- Sensitive/Emotional
- Severe Urges To Drink
- Vomiting/Nausea

Why Withdrawal Occurs

A chronic drinker will experience cravings and withdrawal type symptoms when they initially abstain from alcohol because Alcohol serves as a roadblock to many neural pathways and has an affect on many of the neurotransmitters in the brain. The brain and the body become dependant more and more with the frequency and quantity of use. The predominant effect of alcohol lies in its ability to cause release of gamma aminobutyric acid (GABA)

- Gamma-Aminobutyric acid (GABA) is the chief inhibitory neurotransmitter in the central nervous system. The principal role of GABA is reducing neuronal excitability throughout the nervous system.

Alcohol acts primarily on brain receptors. GABA is the primary inhibitory neurotransmitter in the brain and is the cause of the sedative effects of alcohol. Alcohol, as many other drugs, affects the GABA system just as some prescriptions do, such as antidepressants, sleep aids, anticonvulsants, tranquilizers and muscle relaxants. The euphoric effects of alcohol is due to the increase in dopamine as it is a feel-good hormone. The effects on dopamine are powerful factors in alcohol craving and relapse. Additionally, drinking alcohol interferes with opioid receptors and can lead to a release of beta-endorphins. Beta-endorphins are neuropeptides involved in pain management and they are an endogenous opioid neuropeptide and peptide hormone that is produced in certain neurons within the central nervous system and peripheral nervous system. Alcohol mimics and also inhibits excitatory receptors. Glutamate is the primary excitatory neurotransmitter of the brain, and its inhibition further contributes to the sedative effects of alcohol. Additional important effects on neurotransmitters include increased serotonin activity and decreased nicotinic acetylcholine receptors.

Solutions: Alternative drinks, aminos & supplements, exercise & counselors.

PAWS In longer, more chronic drinkers symptoms can be even worse. The worse withdrawal symptoms can be serious, it is a condition known as delirium tremens (DTs), however, DTs are less common but DTs cause aggressive side effects such as trembling, sweating, confusion, shaking, nausea, vomiting, heart palpitations and even death. After the initial acute withdrawal some will experience PAWS. For those that do experience symptoms, it can last a few days or worst case scenario, for years.

- Aches and Pains
- Craving a Drink
- Depression or Sadness
- Extreme anxiety
- Over emotional and/or no emotion at all
- Persistent Tiredness / Fatigue
- Insomnia / Poor sleep
- Loss of focus / poor concentration
- Memory loss/ poor mental clarity
- Slow cognitive function
- Shakiness/Jitters
- Vertigo/Dizziness/ Off balance

Solutions: Work closely with your counselors, doctors, pastors, mind-body exercises, professionals, use of alternative crutches to replace alcohol.

Length Of Each Phase Of Recovery

Recovery can start. Recovery varies by individual. According to the NIH National Institutes of Health, titled "The Complications of Alcohol Withdrawal", the amount of time it takes to go through detox and alcohol withdrawal depends on each individual and factors like duration, frequency, and heaviness of drinking and symptoms can be mild to severe and life threatening. For most people detox will start about seven hours after the last drink and persist for several days up to a lifetime. For those with severe withdrawal or delirium tremens (DT's) the physical discomfort may last a week or more, and for a few unlucky people protracted withdrawal can last for a year. Alcohol withdrawal can be very mild to very dangerous and medical supervision should be an available option should symptoms become serious.

If you decide to try to do this on your own, you should have friends or family members that you trust to do well checks on you and that you can check in with if a health problem that you can't handle without medical attention should arise. If you are a daily drinker that starts the day out drinking self-detox should never be attempted without medical supervision because it is more likely that you would be more susceptible to medical emergencies, such as seizures, delirium tremens (DT's) and sometimes even death can occur from alcohol withdrawal. About 3% of alcohol withdrawal suffers may experience status-epilepticus (SE's) is a medical emergency that starts when a seizure hits the 5-minute mark, it is rare but it is important to be aware and ready should an emergency SE arise. Substance abuse withdrawal caused by alcohol are often more severe and serious than other drugs because alcohol mimics and hijacks many receptor sites which causes problems such as seizures when neural pathways are blocked from the regulatory effects of neuromodulators and neurotransmitters.

The collection of symptoms known as alcohol withdrawal syndrome (AWS) is from alcohol when it interrupts the brain's mechanism of naturally replacing the neurotransmitters. The exact symptoms, severity, and duration of AWS vary by individual. The longer a person has been drinking, and the more heavily and frequently, the more severe and lasting AWS is likely to be but again there are natural substances and lifestyle changes that will help you through this process. First it is good to know what to expect you may go through this will help you prepare to go through the process so your end result is successful and will help decrease your risk of a relapse.

Endocannabinoid Signaling System

In recent scientific studies, it has been discovered that alcohol drinking and alcohol-preferring behavior are mediated through one of the most abundant neurochemical systems in the central nervous system, the endocannabinoid signaling system. The deletion of CB1 receptors has recently been shown to block voluntary alcohol intake in mice. Mice known to avoid alcohol intake had significantly reduced brain CB1 receptor function. These findings suggest a role for the CB1 receptor gene in excessive alcohol drinking behavior and development of alcoholism in humans. Until then, a broad spectrum hemp supplement may help prevent some of the symptoms of alcohol withdrawal or drinking a tea made of hemp flowers. Additionally, there are physical activities that can increase endocannabinoid signalling besides cannabis or hemp, there are several plants that produce similar therapeutic phyto-cannabinoids including superfoods and common herbs.

8 Common Foods That Contain Phyto-Cannabinoids.

- Black Pepper
- Rosemary
- Kava
- Maca
- Cacao
- Black Truffles
- Echinacea
- Flax seeds

Agmatine is a metabolite of the amino acid arginine. It can help reduce pain, treat drug addiction, and protect the brain from toxins. It has been shown to enhance the painkilling effects of cannabinoids. It does this by increasing cannabinoid action and signalling through the CB1 receptors. My personal experience with agmatine is that it made me agitated, so I stopped taking it but I don't have any symptoms of pain. If you do, I think it's worth trying.

Caryophyllene

Caryophyllene is a compound found in many plants and essential oils, including clove, rosemary, basil, oregano, lavender, and hops. It also contributes to the spiciness of black pepper. Caryophyllene has been shown to have anti-inflammatory, neuroprotective, antidepressant, anti-anxiety and anti-alcoholism effects. These effects are likely because it binds to the cannabinoid receptors. It can also help reduce neuropathic pain through the CB2 receptor.

Dangers of Detox & Alcohol Withdrawal Symptoms

Alcohol detox symptoms will depend on how long you have been dependent on alcohol and how heavily you have drank recently. When you quit, you can expect to suffer with some symptoms called protracted withdrawal syndrome, a condition that may occur after a drinker quits due to sudden or acute withdrawal from alcohol and the symptoms can persist for up to a year. Some people who suffer with PWS experience extended may have symptoms like anxiety, insomnia, tremors, increased heart rate, high blood pressure, temperature fluxuations and labored respiration. Others have symptoms that are opposite of what they experienced in withdrawal such as decreased energy, slowed metabolism, fatigue, and mental weariness. PWS is uncomfortable and because of the discomfort PWS can increase the risk of relapse so awareness, self-care, or ongoing addiction treatment is important.

Delirium tremens usually begins within two to four days of a last drink, but it can occur up to 10 days later. Characteristic symptoms are delirium, which is a sudden type of severe confusion, tremors, agitation, hallucinations, restlessness and bursts of anxious energy, fear, sudden mood changes, deep sleep, and seizures. This dangerous condition is more common in very heavy long term drinkers and of the 5 to 15 % of people who develop delirium tremens die from it. The symptoms of withdrawal typically begin seven to eight hours after a person's last drink. Symptoms may include:

- Delirium
- Tremors/ Shaking
- Light Sensitivity
- Headaches
- Irritation
- Anxiety
- Body Aches
- Joint Pain

- Headache
- Fatigue
- Depression
- Mood swings
- Fight or Flight / Jumpiness
- Difficulty thinking or concentrating
- Nightmares
- Insomnia
- Clammy- chills
- Sweating skin
- Headaches
- Nausea and vomiting
- Decreased appetite
- Cardiac Risk
- Heart Palpitations/Chest pain
- Tremors and shaking
- Moodiness
- Mental Fog
- Cravings
- Seizures
- Death

As you can see, it is a good idea to get a check up from your doctor before you quit and again during the week that you quit.

Delirium Tremens

A dangerous health threat for very heavy, long-term drinkers is an added susceptibility to more serious symptoms of alcohol withdrawal and a condition known as DT's (delirium tremens). Symptoms of DTs may require early medical attention as the symptoms can be dangerous and include fever, hallucinations, agitation, extreme confusion, seizures and death. Call 911 if any signs of DT's arise. The definition of delirium tremens is a psychotic condition involving tremors, hallucinations, anxiety, and disorientation, which alcoholics can suffer from after acute alcohol cessation. The question of "how long does delirium tremens last" is a common question among people who are worried about having it after stopping alcohol consumption. This is sometimes the reason they are afraid to stop. Statistically, DTs occur in 2-5 % of chronic drinkers.

DTs can last just 24 hours for most and five to ten days after the last drink of alcohol for other people. The amount of time generally depends on how long the person has been abusing alcohol and in what amounts. What causes delirium tremens? It is commonly believed that excessive alcohol consumption interferes with the body's ability to regulate the neurotransmitter GABA. The brain starts to mistake alcohol for GABA and limits the production of the neurotransmitter. As the alcohol levels in the body drop, the brain compensates by producing more excitatory neurons (GABA is an inhibitor). The brain then goes into an over excited state, leading to the symptoms described above, as well as further complications, such as seizures. A seizure is usually defined as a sudden alteration of behavior due to a temporary change in the electrical functioning and signaling of the brain. Normally, the brain continuously generates tiny electrical impulses in an orderly pattern. These impulses travel along neurons in the network of nerve cells in the brain and transmitted throughout the whole body via chemical messengers called neurotransmitters. In less than 3% of withdrawal victims seizures may occur and these are usually brief, tonic-clonic type seizures without a preceding aura or headache. This is why amino-acid precursors are a good idea to support the manufacturing of neurotransmitters to lessen the symptoms of withdrawal. This chart illustrates the time of withdrawal with various symptoms.

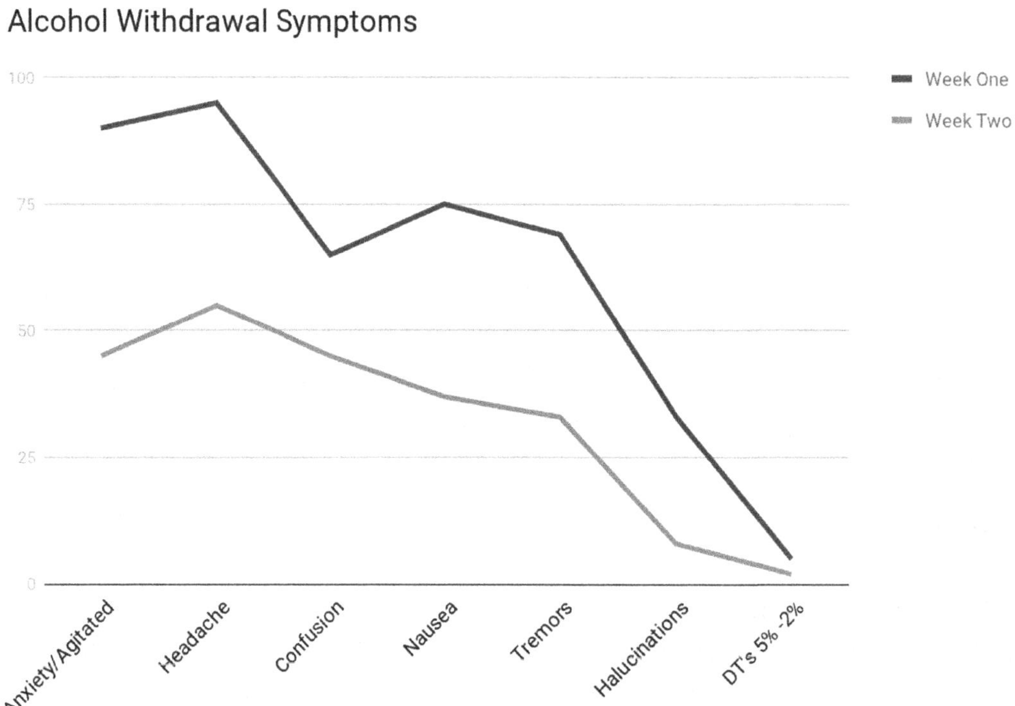

Did I have withdrawal symptoms?

From drinking wine on an almost daily basis for almost three years, yes! Even though I was still considered a light drinker according to the standard charts, when I quit I had some very intense cravings for wine and withdrawal symptoms for several weeks that subsided over time. First of all, I have always been high energy and had a high pain tolerance, before alcohol, I was the kind of person that never gets headaches and rarely ever had the need for pain medication. In the first week of going cold-turkey, I had intense brain fog, I was groggy, it was like I never felt fully awake for a few weeks. My brain felt in a fog without alcohol, the next week my brain literally hurt like a throbbing dull headache, and again I never had headaches, before. Therefore it was a symptom of detox. The 3rd week, i had serious neurological symptoms, I was stone-cold sober, yet, off balance and staggering around like I was drunk and bumping into things while I had been sober for over 3 weeks. For a full month, I was in pain from head down to my toenails. I realized my brain was trying to manufacture the neurotransmitters and my whole body was struggling to start working again on its own, naturally. 6 months after I quit, I had pulsing stabbing headaches in the left posterior brain for days at a time. The only thing that would relieve the headaches was a CBD tincture I formulated for withdrawal. I had unusual pain for over a year as I became use to feeling my body again. I felt like my body was an engine and just as gasoline is ethanol, my body didn't have the fuel to fire all the pistons and cylinders in my brain. It was almost debilitating. At times, I felt almost paralized like I could not move and sometimes when I did I could hardly stand up. I had pain because I could feel my body again off the numbing effects of alcohol. I experienced fatigue, because the pain was exhausting. At times, I had no energy, almost like someone who has a thyroid problem, but in a few months it passed, and I felt like running again.

Quitting With A Weaning Approach

I believe, that by taking a weaning off approach some drinkers will be more successful with less uncomfortable side effects. Alcohol withdrawal is a natural endorphin, hormone and neurotransmitter deficiency syndrome. The last bottle of wine I had in my house was poured down the drain as a freedom from alcohol ritual with my non-drinker best friend. However, in the following weeks my body pain, was so bad once or twice during the first 3 weeks I bought a single serve of shitty twist top wine and took a few small sips and it was awful, I did not enjoy it at all. I poured 1 oz in a dropper bottle, to use as a homeopathic tincture and threw ¾ of it away in the trash where it belonged. If you are a heavy hard liquor drinker, you may pour 1 oz into a gallon of distilled water and take the diluted tincture in place of alcoholic beverages for the first week and in a dropper only drops at a time until withdrawal symptoms are more tolerable. I only took 5 drops twice a day for a week, after that, I eliminated the wine drops and I made and took the same alcohol-free Alcohol-Ease, Quit-Aid and BoozeOff sobriety supplements and tinctures and Quit Brand products, such as Quit-CBD drops and I chewed the kudzu kudchew gum that is sold, today. These products contain powerful natural, nutritional, herbal remedies that have been used for centuries for alcohol withdrawal and detox.

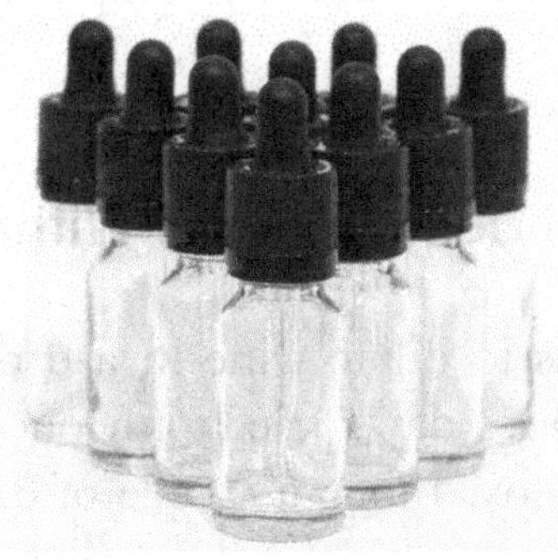

Realizing How Bad Your Alcohol Problem Is

I had went a few days without wine and the symptoms began to show up. I thought so this is what withdrawal feels like. It was the first time I felt pain in years, I was no longer in denial about being a chronic wine drinker, it was obvious my brain neurotransmitters were out of balance. Whenever I would start to do something, it was like I was moving in slow motion as the neurons were not firing properly and all my neural pathways were blocked and in gridlock from being out of fuel. It was an especially disappointing to admit it to myself, with my history that I was somewhat alcohol dependant. Shortly, in the days thereafter, I began to feel deeply again. I felt guilty that I had ever worried my beautiful mother and daughter over my wine drinking. At that moment, I had the realization that wine in fact was trash and that I don't put trash in my body. I also realized that wine had numbed my emotions to the point that I had not felt anything deeply in years. I seldom ever cried, but now the real me was coming back. I felt things. I could feel, again. I felt intense empathy for others. I felt love for my daughter, family, friends and loved ones. I also, began to feel the sting of their words in subtle insults. I was emotionally sensitive. I felt my energy and power coming back. I realized that wine had been robbing me of my power. I could feel my power coming back and the sleeping giant within was beginning to awaken. Then a few days later my whole body, especially my brain was throbbing, pulsing, I wouldn't call it pain but a weird throbbing sensation, all the nerves were coming back to life. This phase was followed by a feeling of being emotionally flat, I didn't feel excited by things that usually excite me. I didnt feel anything remotely resembling excitement or fun. That's when I started taking the amino acids and it helped tremendously. It was the food that my body needed to produce the fuel for manufacturing neurotransmitters, again. A couple of times I had a weird headache and jerking which I feel may have been mild seizures but not enough to be overly concerned. I drank hot cocoa, chamomile and echinacea tea and took other forms of CBD, it all seemed to help and I never had that symptom, again. However, seizure is a serious signal to seek medical attention.

Seizure Risk

Alcohol withdrawal may disrupt the electrical activity of the nervous system and may cause seizures in some individuals that is why it is important to see your doctor prior to quitting and keep them on standby should any complications arise during your Alcohol detox.

Homeopathic Alcohol Dose In Acute Withdrawal

An old folklore remedy was to dilute wine in a dropper bottle and administer 10 drops under the tongue 3-4 times a day. I tried, only once or twice but some say it works well within the first week of detox. I took a couple of drops of wine, from the dropper bottle, when I had a shooting stabbing pain in the nerves in my leg and foot and my brain was throbbing from withdrawal. I didn't even want to use a homeopathic dose of wine at that point, so my best friend gave me a bottle of CBD. I tried it and within minutes my brain was not pulsing or throbbing and I felt normal for the first time since abstaining from alcohol. I formulated a recipe and made my first Quit-Aid and Alco-Ease tincture, which are available online and CBD oil. It worked great to ease all my symptoms and I weaned myself off wine, this way. These were some of my own detox symptoms:

Physical Detox Symptoms:

- Neurotransmitter Imbalance
- Sweating - Hot
- Chills - Cold
- Shaking - Nerves
- Anxiety - Withdrawal Jitters/shakes
- Loss of Balance/Vertigo/Staggering
- Nausea/Vomiting/Stomach Acid
- Insomnia/Restlessness
- Disorientation/Mental Fog
- Malaise - Depressed feeling
- Fatigue - Tired
- Headaches/Brain aches/ Throbbing Head Pain
- Sighing/Rapid breathing
- Body Aches - Pain
- Heart Palpitations
- Cravings - sugar, fruit juice, alcohol, sweets
- Overly Emotional - Sensitive/Crying
- Impatience - Frustration/Easily Agitated
- Sexual dysfunction, loss of desire
- Slow memory recall

I had random ice pick headaches which are classified as a primary stabbing headache. Primary stabbing headaches are caused by overactivity or problems with pain-sensitive structures in the brain. I had some tough days of withdrawal pains and I was tempted to have a drink just to make the pain go away. I know that it was difficult to find incentives to quit and stay sober because it had become such a casual part of my life and I enjoyed the taste of wine. It took more than will power and a desire to quit drinking alcohol and to actually stop. It was uncomfortable but not impossible. I never drank to the point that it caused me serious problems. Although, I drank wine in moderation it was hard to quit. Hopefully, you don't wait until your drinking causes you a heart attack or like many other drinkers, legal problems from DUI's and worse. Don't wait until your drinking becomes a risk of life or death for yourself and others.

Is It Safe To Quit Cold Turkey

It is more safe to quit than it is to continue drinking but for chronic drinkers quit with caution and support through the withdrawal processes. Some drinkers will need help in quitting, but for most people, yes, you can quit safely on your own. Some drinkers will require rehab as some people seem to have worse symptoms than others.

Rehab Options

More addictive type of personality than others and for some it will take more than a 12-step program for them to have success with rehab and long term sobriety. There are a variety of rehab options, like there are many varieties of onions, red onion, sweet onion, green onions, white onions there is no one size fits all in rehab options. What works for one person may not work for another, never quit, never give up keep searching until you find which onion suits your taste and find the rehab plan that works for you.

Alcohol Treatment is Like An Onion With Many Layers And Varieties Of Recovery

Also, after rehab, sometimes the drinker will need to be completely removed from their old drinking environment. Drinkers have to make new non-drinking friends. You will not be successful with your sobriety for very long, if your hanging out at the bar with your old drinking buddies. Its sad but yes, sometimes you have to let people go, too. One rehab approach may not work but another one will. Each person must deal with their struggle on a daily basis. To move-on past your own to have success at healing and recovering.

Myopathy, Nerve Damage and Muscle Wasting

People often drink to relax stiff tight muscles or to calm their nerves, but eventually it damages muscle tone and even nerves. Myopathy is when muscles have wasted and become weak. Muscle weakness is the most frequent symptom of alcoholic myopathy. 40 to 60 % of alcoholics suffer from alcohol-related myopathy. Myopathy can be crippling, causing difficulties in gait, walking, standing from sitting in a chair or in climbing up stairs. In alcoholic myopathy, improvement of muscle weakness usually occurs six to nine months following alcohol abstinence.

Alcohol Sabotages Weight Loss

Alcohol packs on the calories and the pounds. Alcohol affects each person's health in many ways. For me one of the most destructive aspects is that alcohol wrecks a healthy diet. A bottle of wine packs on an extra 700 calories that means you have to run 5.5 miles per hour to burn approximately 740 calories in 60 minutes. For me, I realized that even if I only drank a few sips of wine it would trigger me to eat snacks when I wasn't even hungry. I am sure it is possible for some drinkers that alcohol could trigger cravings for other substances or drugs, like alcohol triggers food cravings for me. One bad habit perpetuates another in a vicious cycle. Bars serve salty snack mix to increase drink sales. As far as drinking and snacking, both are extra between meal calories that will sabotage your health and wreck any weight loss plan.Personally, I realized to be a success at weight loss that I had to quit drinking wine. When I quit I needed something with less calories to substitute the wine, I chose Kombucha tea and snack replacements for my salty peanut carb cravings, I replaced with fruit, celery sticks and raw veggies.

Alcohol As Pain Medicine

I had been hit as a pedestrian and the pain was so intense for the first few months I could not sleep at night. Everyone, knows there is an Opiate abuse and pain pill addiction epidemic, so, I refused the narcotic pain meds the doctor offered me and even with the anti-inflammatory medications, my knee injury would burn with intense pain, constantly. I was in pain from the accident and I was tempted to drink alcohol as a pain reliever but opted out for CBD oil and chiropractic, it worked. I also tried hyperbaric oxygen chamber therapy that is the therapy the professional orthopedics for pro athletes when they get injured. HBO therapy helps speed recovery of injuries without drugs or surgery as it helps the body produce stem cells to repair the injuries in the body. When you start your rehab it is likely you will experience body pain. Alcohol numbs your physical pain and emotional pain. The pain is a sign you are and your body are learning to feel, again. You may be tempted to relapse if the pain is too great, take a normal dose of over the counter pain reliever as directed on the manufacturer label to prevent this from spoiling your recovery and sobriety and talk to a counselor that can help you deal with emotional pain in a healthy manner.

Chapter 12

Healing Painful Emotions As Relapse Prevention

Emotional Pain During Detox and Rehab

The tears may come from years of repressed emotions. It is normal, and yes this part of recovery and yes, for a little while it may hurt like hell. Keep in mind that alcohol has been your emotional crutch for quite a while, for some, for years, maybe even since childhood. If we take a closer look at our alcohol use, we find that the feelings that drive us to drink are the ones that most go to great measures to avoid suffering those same emotions that have been suppressed by alcohol use. Those painful emotions that trigger substance abuse can trigger relapse. It is pain and the fear of pain, be it physical, emotional, mental or psychological that drives us to mind altering forms of substance abuse. Part of recovery is learning NOT to drink away the tears and instead of developing better interpersonal skills and learning to openly express your emotions and feelings in a healthy manner.

Ghost From The Past During Alcohol Withdrawal

As we sober up, we may become very sensitive to feelings and emotions, like a tender hearted child. Many of the past emotional traumas you may have experienced and all the tears you swallowed with alcohol may be exhumed. As children, when we cried, many of us were told to suck it up and dry it up by our care-givers or even mocked and called a "cry-baby" by siblings or other children. Hurt feelings and emotions are going to come up during rehab, without the alcohol-crutch to make us feel emotionally numb, you may become hyper-sensitive for a short period. It is ok to cry. In fact, it is good to cry. The average human cries 10 gallons of tears in an average lifetime. Crying is a healthy means of releasing psychological grief and sadness. Cry and get all those old emotional wounds out to release them and let them go, forever. Part of successful recovery and lifelong sobriety is understanding what drives our behavior to drink so that we are not tempted to self-medicate. Crying helps us heal. If the pain feels too much, you don't have to suffer through it alone, you can confide in a trusted friend or seek the advice of a professional counselor. If you experienced childhood abuse, it is best not to do these exercises alone, seek professional help, first.

Importance Of Journaling

Journaling is your chance to write down all your thoughts and feelings and get them out of your head on paper. Journaling is proven to help process pent up thoughts, feelings and emotions. There is an "I Quit" journal that can be purchased separately as an adjunct to this book. It is an alcohol rehab workbook that offers additional success tips and solutions for a successful sober lifestyle. The "I Quit" journal is filled with lots of space to track your progress or you can journal in any notebook. You can practice writing your self-medicating drinking story, here:

Self-Medicating Prevention Journaling Exercise
My Life Story of Hurts And Wounds

This is an example of mine:

When I was a child, I was a hyper-inquisitive child out of five of us siblings and I was probably a little too overwhelming for my mom, who was a very passive personalities person. For some reason, I "worried her" and "got-on'her-nerves" I asked mom why and she said "that I could never sit still and I was always into something" which is true, once I when I was 4 or 5 years old, I overdosed on baby aspirins and then another time on cough syrup and had to have my stomach pumped. I had to have stitches a couple of times too, so my dad was appointed to keep an eye on me. I spent most of our spare time hanging out with my dad, his name was Pete, he was outgoing and had many friends, he was ex-military and trained as a mechanical engineer, after discharge he got a job as a mechanic supervisor at a conveyor belt manufacturer. Dad had a hobby, he was a breeder of pedigree walker hound dogs and he trained and sold them on the side, so we always had lots of animals, once we had 26 puppies. I think that is one reason why dogs have always been a sort of emotional support pet for me. Dad bought me my first bike, a glittery blue banana seat bike with white pom-poms and a white basket. He bought my first pony, a solid white grey horse I named "Tom" he spent hours teaching me how to properly take care of "Tom". Dad was the best and he knew how to keep me busy and happy! He was my best friend. I use to annoy my mom and older siblings asking too many questions but dad never let me down, if I had a question he was always available to answer it, even when he wasn't home I could call him on the phone. I was his shadow, he took me with him almost everywhere, I would help him feed and groom the dogs, and fetch his tools for him whenever he was working on something around the farm and people would call us Pete and re-Pete after the older siblings were grown and left home, I felt even closer to dad. Sadly, dad died suddenly when he was only 39 years old in a tragic auto accident. I was only 10 years old. My mom was traumatized and had to work extra to support me and my little sister, alone as a widowed mom. In those days, in the south, the adults in my life, would say, your dad is in heaven with god. I never had grief counseling until I was an adult. I was angry that my dad had died and left us, one day, I could not be consoled and threw a rather dramatic emotional outburst of grief that my mom was unprepared to deal with. My flood of emotional grief overwhelmed her. After a few hours, she said, you will see your daddy again, in heaven. I remember missing my dad so badly that I wanted to die, so I could go see him, in heaven. My mom said, "I know your upset, we all miss your dad, but you have to accept that your dad is gone and he's never coming back and we can't go see him so stop crying and acting out like this or we will have to go to the hospital and the doctors there keep people who act like this in the insane asylum. I asked where is that and she said, they send crazy people to the insane asylum and keep them until they can act normal". I was also a very active, outdoor kid I loved riding my bike and horse around the loop my dad built on our 65 acre homeplace, I was a nature lover and an animal lover, and not only did I lose my dad when he died, but because we couldn't take care of the animals without dad, my mom sold my horse and dad's dogs. Additionally, we moved away from the 65 acre farm into a house closer to moms work and switched schools and I lost my cat, Thomasina, during that move. All of my emotional support animals were gone. The following year, my mom bought me a german shepherd, I named him razor, he was my emotional support animal.

Emotional Drinking Similar To Emotional Eating

By doing this journaling exercise, you may find many emotional triggers related to your drinking. Especially, females who are careful to watch what they eat to stay slim, may resort to emotional drinking over emotional eating. I believe if we can have an emotional eating disorder we can also have an emotional drinking disorder. I experienced several childhood woundings and drastic changes within a year of my father's passing. I kept my grief inside, I repressed my emotions and turned my attention to music. I joined the band and focused on music, learning to play several instruments and wrote songs and poems and kept a diary, my friends became my therapy I was voted class favorite 3 years in a row and strived for excellence in academics and music and mom was proud. I progressed on to becoming a majorette and focused on keeping my body fit, to look good in my majorette costumes. I can remember being obsessed with weight loss and keeping my body in shape. That's another reason why I became a fitness trainer and then a nutritionist, too. I had emotional eating issues that I overcame with fitness training and the wine use was an alternative to an emotional eating, I began, emotional drinking.

It wasn't until years later that I realized it is not about what your eating or drinking, it's about what's eating you that your trying to drown with booze. Getting into healthcare and wellness allowed me a safe place, that I felt safe enough to finally be able to release all those tears of grief. As it turned out, I carried the repressed emotions and my dad's ghost around with me through most of my life, it was one of the emotions that I was numbing with wine when forgiveness would have ended the pain. We can't change the past but we can forgive and forget the grudges we hold against our abusers.There are many alcohol support groups with people going through the same stage of recovery, that can help you through this "crying-stage" of recovery in a safe, supportive setting. Use the following quiz form to get in touch with any past abuse, neglect or crying triggers to bring awareness to your emotional triggers and to help avoid self-medicating your emotional pain and suppressed tears or repressed emotions with alcohol. You can practice writing your drinking trigger abuse or neglect story, here:

Who Abused Me And Who Protected Me As A Child Or Adult

____

____

Today, I forgive and forget this gruge I hold against my abuser: ________________

____

____ Date: ____________

Here is an example of my self-work quiz:

> After my dad died, I remember missing my mom while she had to work and support me and my younger sibling, as a single mom, after my dad died. I remember being hungry and missing my parents. Our babysitter was a tyrant who was angry all the time. I remember being yelled and screamed at by the babysitter and ordered to do things I didn't want to do instead of doing my homework. I was kicked, hit, slapped, and on one occasion while trying to take an encyclopedia to read out of the parlor the babysitter kicked me into the door facing and I was knocked unconscious, when I awoke I was in surgery getting stitches on my eye. The babysitter said it was an accident, and I kept quite in fear of the babysitter. We had another babysitter, this one was almost as abusive but better, still I remember being made to do the work of a maid as a teenager. I remember being held down and choked because I wore my bathing suit out of the house in public view. I was bullied and screamed at by the babysitter on a continual constant daily basis. I couldn't wait to get old enough to drive so we wouldn't need a babysitter. As soon as I turned 15, I got my drivers permit and worked a summertime job to raise money for a car. I got my drivers license on the day I turned 16 and my mom bought my first car. I became responsible for taking my little sister to school and picking her up. I drove us to band practice and myself to state college for half the school day. I did this for 2 years. I found myself left in an empty home with my little sister in the evenings and often she turned her anger and

disappointment toward me on a few occasions and being a badly wounded child, myself, I was not mature enough or capable of dealing with her emotions regarding our situation because I was traumatized, myself. I took my little sister and myself to school at 7:15 am, left high school at lunch drove to state community college in a neighboring town got out at 3, drove back to the high school for band practice till 7 drove home and did homework with my sister and washed dishes and got our school clothes ready for the next day before bedtime. At some point, my older brother and his wife moved into our new house and I remember coming in after 9 pm and I had twirled and marched in my senior homecoming parade and I was exhausted but still forced to wash all their dishes for the whole household when I wasn't even there to eat and I was forced to do all the dirty laundry for the whole family too. There is a difference in having children to do chores to pickup after themselves, but using them as a maid, is slavery. My mom really didn't know how we were being treated while she was at work, I began coming home later and later to avoid being yelled at and used as a slave and by the weekend mom was tired so every saturday morning, I would do her work clothes laundry for her and I remember being scolded for not drying the clothes properly or separating the clothes properly but I tried my best to help her. I felt in despair and left home the day I turned 18. I never received any support from my parents again until the last 3 years of my mom's life and it was one of the most healing processes we ever experienced, together.

Today, I forgive and forget this grudge I have held against: _

I forgive my mom for neglecting some of my childhood needs after the loss of my dad, I understand mom was struggling from loss issues, too and was heavily burdened and stressed as a single mom.I believe she trusted those whom she relinquishcd my care to do no harm to me in her absence. I forgive my babysitters for abusing me and for mistreating me. I accept that I can't change the past or the evil deeds of others. I release my rage and pain and I put their judgement in gods hands to deal with them. I am now free from them. I claim my happiness, joy and success. Amen

Date:4/20/2010

If you have issues with your parents, babysitters or other caregivers, it is a good idea to go to a family therapist, together. I didn't have the chance with my mom until her retirement, since my father died because she was in survival mode from the day my dad died until her kids moved out and she retired. It was very healing to have the chance to heal my childhood wounds with her and made me very happy to work through my past childhood traumas by spending a lot of time with my elderly mother. From 2010 till 2014

I traveled back to see her and spend time with her every few weeks and I can say, we talked about it all, everything and together we healed our relationship together. I loved my mom and she loved me and we had a special bond through music. My mom made up for everything in the end we had a very loving close bond and understanding of each other.

Repressed grief abuse and being parentized as a child was a deep emotional trauma that when I was in my 30's began to surface and I numbed with wine until my mom and I could work through the painful past together and resolve my feelings of being neglected as a child although my mom was a great mom, feeling that she didn't protect me from other abusive caregivers was an issue that was unresolved and unforgiven for many years. However, I had other unresolved issues, too. I always had a respect for my mother and I never drank in front of my mother. After, doing most of the wellness treatments in this book, I was able to give up drinking because those old wounds wasn't a trigger anymore.

Parentizing Children Causative Factors In Alcoholism

Parentizing children is an intergenerational relational pattern that is the most common cause of adult codependency and involves something known as the reversal process. In reversal processes parents or other caregiving adults place their duties on children with high expectations above their capabilities and maturity level. A child becomes parentatized by having to take on adult responsibilities within the household or when an adult gives children too many adult responsibilities or use children to meet their own needs causing emotional, psychological and performance stress resulting in potentially long term post traumatic stress and anxiety in adulthood. It is similar to surrogate spouse parenting, there are many ways parents and caregivers can wound children. Many people have childhood traumas that may drive them to drug abuse in adulthood so it is important to heal by working with a counselor.

Childhood "Emotional Wounding"

The shadow self forms, usually in childhood, over some painful emotional wounding trauma. Usually, childhood wounding occurs when some situation that our feelings were not treated as being important or when we did not feel loved enough or we felt hurt or devalued as a person. Children are tender hearted and emotionally sensitive, they are like a sponge soaking up information that helps form their personality, all while making a blueprint for how to give and receive love. Children learn to live their life by example from the adult role-models around them. A child's personality develops between birth and around 5 years old. A child learns their reason, logic and decision making skills between 8-12 usually by observing how their primary caregiver relates and negotiates with their primary caregiver. If we are not supported properly through these stages of growth we can develop self-esteem issues. When we are emotionally traumatized, hurt or shamed, as a child, we make a contract with ourselves to never allow anyone to hurt us like that again. By making this contract or promise to our child-self, we build a psychological protective barrier around ourselves to prevent anything similar from ever hurting us again. Sometimes, people even have amnesia regarding their childhood wounding, so you may not remember it. Our body's self-healing, if you cut yourself within days the scab falls off and we have new skin underneath. The mind is different, mental and emotional wounds, our coping mechanisms may cause amnesia or kind of build a mental brick wall around our heart and memories. It is there, where your shadow self is born, it is the part of us that will get ugly if we feel threatened, it may even cause a person to develop a character flaw, such as dishonesty. It sets a pattern of ignoring emotions early on and then people start drinking alcohol to cope with emotions later on.

For example, if when you were 5 years old, your mom told you she was taking you to the zoo and then to get ice cream. You jumped for joy, ran to get your shoes on, with a big smile on you face, you happily got in the car and was bouncing up and down with excitement as you jabbered on about the animals you couldn't wait to see at the zoo, but then you arrive, get out to find, mom had took you to the dentist to get your tooth pulled, you went through an unexpected emotional trauma filled with disappointment, fear, tears, anger and pain but then in the end the child got an ice pack for a sore bleeding mouth and an ice cream but then went to the zoo and later she told you to put your pulled tooth under your pillow for the tooth fairy to come creeping into your bed at night to exchange it for a quarter, WTH!!! This is obviously deceptive parenting and quite barbaric by today's standards. Since children learn by example, those types of scenarios teach the child it's ok to manipulate others to get them to do what you want, and it teaches them it's ok to lie. The only thing telling children the tooth fairy and santa clause, is it teaches the child is to lie and have a lack integrity. The parent may think they are saving their child and themself some stress on the way to the dentist but by keeping their child from crying, pitching a fit or refusing to go to the dentist just denies the child the opportunity to express their emotions honestly and openly. Some abusive parents may even take it a step further and scold or spank their child for acting up at the dentist, or may verbally belittle their child by calling them a cry-baby or other insulting names. Later as an adult the child inside won't know how express their true feelings, ither. It may have saved the parent some stress while driving to the dentist but it was still a wounding experience for a child that will be carried into adulthood and perhaps, for the rest of their life. The child will always have issues with honesty and integrity. As an adult they will lie and manipulate. The truth is always the best parenting method. Parents do not realize how their actions affect their children's personality or may cause character flaws and usually it is not intentional it comes from poor parenting skills and lack of child development psychology knowledge but there are many other negative characteristics that could develop over these types of emotional woundings or trust betrayals in childhood and one of them is substance abuse in adulthood. The shadow-self is the part of yourself that you hide from the rest of the world. The shadow self is often irrational because it is a child's thoughts. In this example, it's the 5 year old subconscious mind programming, saying, I will never trust another woman to take me to the zoo or anywhere, for the rest of my life! Unfortunately, it is the part that will keep sabotaging the opportunity to have all the good things in life. Because, somewhere deep inside that wounded inner child was taught to believe that something is wrong with themself. The shadow self is self destructive and participates in substance abuse. The "wounding-contract" is often irrational and breaking the contract is the key to emotional self healing and ultimately, sobriety. There is only one way to heal those inner injuries and that is by doing your emotional work, having a healthier mindset and learning to live life in a state of forgiveness and love. If you have memories of any type of emotional or physical abuse seek a counselor to help you do your shadow work and encourage you family to see a marriage and family therapist so the healing process can begin.

Pain From Alcohol Detox

One night during the first week of detox, I was in such terrific pain, my whole body hurt and I was having random electric shock like stabbing pains that felt so real, as if I was actually being stabbed. I was not thinking clearly, I had mental fog. I was looking for something to ease the pain, but I was out of over-the-counter ibuprofen. This is the stage of detox when many addicts and alcohol abusers accidentally overdose. In a brain fog, I found an old prescription of 800 mg. Ibuprofen that my dentist had prescribed and I took 2 because my body pain was so great that I could not sleep. It made me very nauseated, then I had a mild cardiac arrhythmia so I took my heart miracle remedy and my heart settled down to normal rhythm. I made sure I was hydrated, drank enough distilled water. The next day, I switched to over the counter ibuprofen it helped enough with the pain while I researched what I could take that was natural to facilitate my detox as my body started producing its own endorphins and neurotransmitters again. I discovered some effective, alternatives that may work for you too, as a relapse preventative. The list of natural remedies are in the dietary supplement section of this book. If you have a dual diagnosis, such as taking and being dependant on prescription pain medications, in addition to alcohol use, please, see your health provider for medical care and help to ease you through this stage of recovery, safely.

About Assisted Alcoholism Rehab

Alcoholism is the worst stage of alcohol abuse. 1-5% of Alcohol abusers will need institutionalized rehab as the withdrawal can become so intense that is becomes dangerous. There are many options, I believe the most effective approach is an integrative medical alcohol rehab program that includes mind body therapies and exercise. Choose a treatment center that offers therapy that provide hope by making you understand that you can make positive changes in your life and empowers you with the belief in your ability to recover. The therapy allows you to improve your well-being and health while addressing emotional challenges, trauma or mental health disorders that may have contributed to addiction. All programs are designed to give you access to recovery tools that aren't available to alcoholics who sober up without treatment.

Through detox, counseling, group therapy, medication or dietary supplement therapy and recovery education, you will learn how to best manage your sobriety. DT's are a risk for the chronic disease of alcoholism. The resources you'll gain in rehab include:

- An understanding of the nature of your own alcoholism
- The triggers, causes and the roots of your addiction
- Coping skills for avoiding a slip or for reducing risk of relapse
- A stronger sense of purpose and self-esteem
- Stronger relationships with loved ones, family, friends and employers
- A deeper knowledge of how alcoholism affects your physical and emotional health
- An awareness of how staying sober enhances your life
- How being sober helps you reach your full potential
- A happier and healthier future of sobriety.

Rehab programs should offer a full range of services, including individual therapy, peer support groups, pharmacotherapy, treatment of any underlying or co-occurring mental health conditions and holistic therapies. The more tools you have at your disposal, the more likely you are to feel engaged in sobriety.

Sobriety And Emotional Health

One of the most important reasons to address negative emotions and to learn to control or manage them is to manage triggers and avoid relapsing. Negative feelings are often triggers for substance use, and if they are not regulated a relapse becomes nearly inevitable. The less obvious reason to work toward emotional sobriety is that it improves overall mental health and quality of life. Emotional sobriety is a concept that originated with Alcoholics Anonymous the 12-step method, a support group program for those who struggle with drinking. Participants work through the steps to achieve lasting sobriety. The final step requires taking the message to others, while also living the steps and practicing principles in everything a person does and that those who have completed the program should help others achieve it. Emotional sobriety is complicated and difficult to define, but generally it means being able to experience, confront, and accept all emotions, even the painful ones. It doesn't mean being happy all the time, but it does mean having a healthy relationship with emotions and using positive strategies to cope with those that are negative. It is a complex and long process to learn to become emotionally sober.

Sobriety Success Support Action Plan

Even if you remain friends with those who drink, it can help to have sober friends as a separate support system. Try meeting sober friends through health conscious activities, like volleyball, hiking, church retreats, wellness retreats, a sober living meetup, yoga class, rehab alumni group, a 12-step meeting or another sober environment. Also, suggest some sober activities to your drinking friends so your encounters don't always involve alcohol. For example, try a nature activity, engage in an exercise class or sport, or join a class to learn a hobby.

an outpatient treatment program can provide strategies for moving forward with life in recovery, including how to handle triggers and temptations. Also, an aftercare program and 12-step meetings can provide continuing support after rehab to make it easier to avoid relapse and stick with recovery.

Tips on Sobriety Around Friends Who Drink

The hardest part is going back out into the social scene with your friends, family or colleagues whom you may have went out drinking with in the past before your sobriety. The following examples may work for you when socializing with your old drinking buddies without having to make the whole social event a never ending stream of explanations.

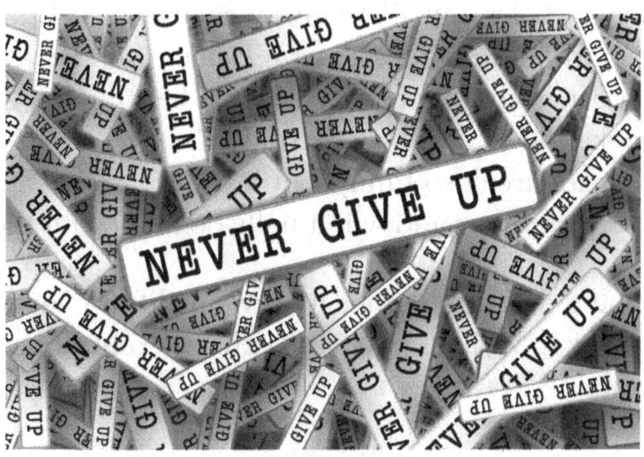

ON YOUR SOBRIETY

Make a Joke

As I write this for you, today it is April 1st, or April Fool's Day. I wish I could tell you something that would motivate you enough to guarantee your permanent lifelong sobriety success.

Sobriety Makes You Rich & Sexy!

Just kidding! Hey, but like those weight loss reality TV shows where you win a million dollars if you lose the most weight, something has to keep you motivated after the contest and the money's gone. Sobriety won't make you rich but quitting drinking does make you look healthier and feel better and it will give you a better chance in life at becoming rich and successful more than becoming an alcoholic will. Sobriety is a much better option over being an alcoholic your whole life. Alcohol robs you of your full potential in life. If sobriety made us rich and alcoholism makes us poor then neither one of us would have never picked up that first drink. Sobriety does make us sexier and that is true, just look at some before and after photos of people who quit drinking. They are always better looking in the after photos. There is nothing sexy about being a sloppy drunk, so yes, sobriety makes you sexier! Use humor while turning down someone who offers to buy you a drink. Humor is always a good way to turn someone's drink offer down without making their kindness feel rejected. Say something like:

1. Nice of you to offer, but, I'm trying to keep both feet on the ground, tonight's not the night for me to get falling down drunk, but hey lets dance!
2. "No thanks buddy, at this point, I'm still conscious, better not add vodka to the mix.
3. Thanks darling, but, "I'm driving and not keen on sleeping if off in a drunk cell tonight also I look horrible in stripes."
4. Awh thanks for the offer, but, I'm clumsy enough as it is and since I'm driving tonight better not risk stumbling around if I should wind up in a field sobriety test.
5. No thanks, I'm driving and not really keen on becoming a gang bang toy for the boys in cell block B down at the po-po station.
6. Sure, sarcastic jokes aren't so funny, but it could also help your friend to take a reality check for themselves and will usually do away with the drink offers.

If someone buys you a drink and sends it over, just lift up your class and say cheers then do not actually drink it, without having to explain. Your not obliged to explain, it's your choice not to drink.

Take Time For Simple Pleasures And Joys

- Keep a Gratitude journal
- Drink hot tea and have a good convo
- Perform a random act of kindness
- Play with a puppy or kitten
- Go for a jog / Power Walk
- Volunteer to help someone
- Meditate or Pray
- Go on a Vacation
- Take a hand in hand walk
- Smile
- Laugh
- Exchange Massages
- Make Love
- Take a Nap

Break The Vicious Cycle

Educate yourself on the long term outcomes of including alcohol in your lifestyle. The longer you drink alcohol, the harder it becomes to quit and the more you will need to drink to get the same effect. You will build up a tolerance and dependency will begin to require greater quantities to feel the effect and as you drink more and more to get the same feeling the more your body and brain will suffer damage and respond by producing less neurotransmitters, eventually, you will become an alcoholic, your brain will stop producing enough neurotransmitters on its own and then your body can not function without having a drink, eventually, it becomes a vicious cycle of alcohol dependence.

Each person varies in their own tolerance. The longer you drink alcohol, the harder it becomes to quit and the more you drink, the worse you feel in the hangover phase. Alcohol causes depression, loss of motivation, impaired coordination, difficulty walking, blurred vision, slurred speech, slowed reaction times, impaired memory. Clearly, alcohol negatively affects the brain. Some impairments are temporary while others are permanent. Impairment is detectable after only one drink. There are newly proposed government mandates to lower the legal blood alcohol lower than what it is. After two alcohol beverages impairment is evident. However, impairments quickly resolve when drinking stops and you can do treatments to repair the damage that was caused from alcohol. However, chronic daily drinking is accumulative and may cause continual impairments. Heavy binge drinking can result in permanent liver and brain damage and also can cause permanent damage to the nervous system.

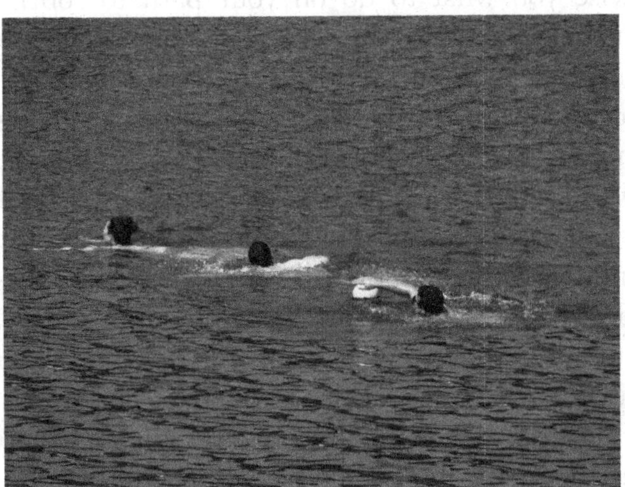

Health Recovery After Alcohol Abuse

The initial first step to health recovery after alcohol abuse is an awareness assessment to determine how deep of a situation you are in with alcohol. If you are a light to moderate drinker or if you are a heavy drinker or alcoholic. If you are a light to moderate drinker you can most likely abstain or quit drinking alcohol on your own, without some serious complications from the withdrawal. However, if your a heavy drinker, you may be at risk for medical complications or if you are an alcoholic you will need medical assistance through the first week or so of detox to monitor any life threatening symptoms.

Abstaining From Alcohol Think Safety 1st

The second step is to detox your body. Detoxification cleanses the toxins from your cells and organs and helps them regain their normal functioning. The next phase, is adopt a healthy diet and sobriety lifestyle and the final stage is to have lots of stick-to-it-ivness. Many light drinkers who use alcohol occasionally and who are not over-drinkers, can simply quit drinking and many of their problems will disappear. Some people who drink regularly who are light to moderate drinkers will also be able to quit on their own. However, heavy alcoholics will need more professional help in quitting safety and it is always a good idea to have a medical checkup and medical attention plan, in case something goes wrong during transitioning through dangerous and sometimes fatal DT's. If you are an alcoholic, plan your medical assistance beforehand, from the beginning of your drinking cessation plan. After the first few weeks you will be in a better position to safely do more self-care as you transition into a sobriety lifestyle.

Medical Check Up

Anyone can advise you what to do on your path to sobriety but you have to incorporate, tips and methods into your lifestyle. Ultimately, you will do the work yourself. Still having a medical check up before, during and after the initial detox phase is wise. Supervision is key to safe alcoholism detox. Although there are natural remedies to use at home to ease alcohol withdrawal symptoms, detoxing from alcohol or any other drug. Men as well as women should abstain from alcohol for at least three months prior to conception to ensure a healthy baby free from the effects of alcohol fetal syndrome, learning disabilities and birth defects. For Pregnant or lactating women, methods of alcohol detox is always to be determined by their doctor and obviously if you are pregnant or lactating you should not be drinking alcohol for any reason. Alcohol fetal syndrome is seriously dangerous for developing babies. The smallest amount will pass through into mothers milk as well. If you are a drinker, do not get pregnant until you are alcohol free, if you are a nursing mother, do not drink alcohol and if you plan to have a drink it is better to bottle feed your baby for at least 32 hours after you've had a drink. Parents also set a role model example for children so it's also important not to set the example of drinking alcohol. Children of addicts are eight times more likely to develop an addiction. A 1985 study suggests a strong genetic component, particularly for the onset of alcoholism in males. Generally, if parents use drugs, sooner or later their children will as well.

Alcohol Abstinence

While cutting back on alcohol consumption is a good idea, but honestly, it rarely works, the idea is one binge away from total failure and becoming abstinent from alcohol is the only real solution, that will certainly improve every ex-drinker's health greatly. Sobriety will not remove the psychological issues an ex-drinker struggles with. For instance, if you were using alcohol as a self-medication for anxiety, the anxiety issue is likely to flare up, a doctor can help you with an appropriate anxiety management and it is not always going to require medication.

The National Institutes of Health (NIH) suggests that recovery from alcohol abuse depends on many factors, such as:

- Dependance- How long the individual abused alcohol
- Tolerance- the amount of alcohol used/abused
- Genetics- A person's and genetic makeup
- Family history- alcoholic relative
- Lifestyle factors- health, diet, exercise, habits, etc.
- Mental Health- psychiatric, cognitive, social
- Physical Health- medical conditions that are co-occurring with alcohol use disorders

Ultimately, chronic use and alcohol abuse may be associated with other comorbid conditions, medical conditions, neurological conditions, psychological conditions, and social issues all considered medical issues.

Addiction Is A Physical As Well as a Mental Problem

Abstaining from alcohol use can help in most of these issues improving but continuing to use alcohol will only result in these issues being exacerbated. Individuals who suffer from illnesses related to their use of alcohol should quit and if they can't do it on their own without risk the can seek professional treatment for both their alcohol use and any other related conditions.

Liver Recovery After Alcohol Damage

The liver is one of the most complex organs in the human body and alcohol destroys it but there is good news, too. Even if you had 75 % of your liver removed it can grow back to its full size and there is even more good news when it comes to repairing your liver, by abstaining from drinking alcohol drinking lots of water, and eating a liver-friendly diet and a few simple at home self-care liver remedies, you can often reverse some of the effects of alcohol abuse. The liver can repair itself after years of drinking with its incredible function of filtering toxins out of the body, in fact the liver has over 500 functions. These include filtering out blood toxins, storing energy, making hormones and proteins, regulating cholesterol and blood sugar. Alcoholic liver disease is a result of over consuming alcohol that damages the liver, leading to a buildup of fats, inflammation, and scarring. It can be fatal. The condition is a primary cause of chronic liver disease in the U.S.

Damaging Effects Of Ethanol Metabolism On The Liver

When ingested orally, ethanol alcohol is extensively metabolized by the liver. Our liver metabolizes the ethanol in alcoholic drinks thanks to the enzyme alcohol dehydrogenase. Ethanol alcohol robs and depletes the liver of enzymes. Ethyl Alcohol increases the secretion of acids in the stomach. The metabolite acetaldehyde is responsible for much of the short term, and long term effects of ethyl alcohol toxicity that is so damaging to your liver. There are many ways to help your liver recover after alcohol abuse but don't wait until you drink your liver and cirrhosis, cancer or hepatitis before you quit drinking and start help your liver recover. Some alcohol-related liver damage can be reversed if you stop drinking alcohol early enough before the disease process ensues. Healing can begin as early as a few days to weeks after you stop drinking. However, once alcoholic liver disease progresses, its symptoms become apparent. The distinct signs of late-stage liver diseases include:

- Jaundice and a yellow tint of the whites of the eyes and the skin
- Edema and swelling of the lower limbs
- Ascites/beer belly (buildup of fluid in the abdomen)
- Fever, cold-sweats and shivering
- Itchy skin
- Club fingernails that curve with yellowing
- Weight loss
- Weak or wasting muscles
- Blood in vomit and stools
- Bleeding thinning skin and bruising

Once those symptoms are noticeable, the condition has reached an advanced stage, and visiting a doctor is a crucial next step. People with acute alcoholic hepatitis must be treated in a hospital.

Liver failure can result from alcohol consumption. A liver transplant is a life threatening process and is considered a last resort. Quitting alcohol and treating liver damage or disease early on is the best way for a person to increase their chances of saving their liver and reversing the disease. There are several foods, herbs and spices that strengthen hepatic health and liver function. A good daily drink for liver health is liver detox tea.

FREEDOM IN SOBRIETY

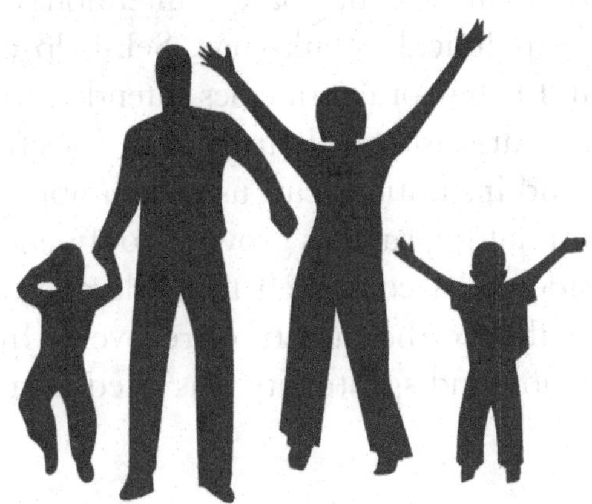

Mental Preparation- Positive Psychology- sounds much like the power of positive thinking, however, it is beyond that. It is important to get yourself psyched up mentally to conquer your addiction to alcohol. Positive psychology uses evidence-based interventions, or positive interventions to filter effective strategies from those that may sound pleasing but fail to enhance well-being. Choice is a large part in developing addiction, but choice disappears with the onset of addiction. In other words, individuals chose to use drugs and/or engage in addictive behaviors until addiction is active, at which point addiction is self-perpetuating. Despite losing volition in active addiction, once drugs and/or behaviors are extinguished for a short time, volition is restored. Addiction is associated with brain circuitry and functional changes that impedes the pursuit of happiness. However, these changes do not prevent addicts from either quitting using addictive substances, engaging in addictive behaviors, or desiring to maximize their well-being. Addicts are motivated to quit by the very same moral and pragmatic, or well-being enhancing, elements that catalyzed their engagement with the disease. Addicts don't quit to minimize their "multifaceted dysfunction," they quit to pursue happiness.

Positive Psychology: is an adjunct therapy to psychology that teaches happiness often requires intentional self-regulation and the development of good habits. According to a review of nine clinical studies, positive psychology, when applied to a substance use, addiction, and recovery program, showed, positive psychological benefits, distinguished from traditional psychology it is a mental health work that is dedicated to reducing suffering and decreasing pathology. Positive psychology is important as a supplement to traditional psychology in an integrative recovery program that emphasizes some important perspectives that have long been under-emphasized and neglected in psychology. For example, long before being labeled "positive psychology" the great philosophers: Socrates, Plato & Aristotle and also, psychological thinkers: Freud, Jung, Adler, Frankl, Rogers, Maslow each articulated theories of living in a positive view of life, creating the good life, finding pleasures in life, wholesomeness in living, finding a purpose, maintaining good physical health, and self actualization.

Success in Spirituality & Positive Recovery

A positive intervention is an evidence-based, intentional act, designed to increase well-being, primarily in non-clinical populations. Self-help considered as simple, self-administered, cognitive and behavioral strategies intended to increase individual well-being. Positive psychology can also be defined as a 'positive' tool that individuals, clinicians, organizations, and institutions can use when appropriate. 'Positive' refers to the better aspects of human nature, such as growth, confidence, resilience, honesty, and integrity. In addition, randomized controlled trials demonstrate that spirituality may reduce relapse rates and enhance the quality of recovery. In one study of recovering addicts, strength from religion and spirituality was cited as a cause of highly favorable outcomes.

Alcoholics Anonymous

There are many treatment and support group options available. Perhaps the most common one is AA, they have helped many people achieve sobriety. You may look into their program and see if it is a fit for you. The Big Book of Alcoholics Anonymous is a 12-Step recovery program that utilizes spirituality and taking a spiritual approach for strength. God is mentioned in 4 of the 12 steps, and being a christian, myself, I like that. Recovery fellowships encourage a noncompetitive approach to life that promotes well-being for its members and unifies them in altruism, kind of like a church support group and approaches life as a life-long recovery program which I don't entirely agree with but it works for many and it may work for you, too. There is more good to agree with in their program than their is to disagree over.

Recovery Maintenance Phase

Recovery consists of these main parts:

1. Sobriety Adherence - commitment to sobriety, doing the things at home and on your own that you've learned to be successful in sobriety for the prevention of relapse
2. Positive Recovery Daily Meditation- rewires the neurons to think like a non-addict, sober mindset. Deeply think or meditate on sober life goals. Vision of life without alcohol.
3. Journal - self-work, write thoughts, feelings, goals & accomplishments.
4. Reinforcement - daily self-intervention and exercising weak areas.
5. Positive psychology- positive and effective lifestyle assistance
6. Join an Online Support Group- recovery support group,

7. Gratitude Exercises- reminders of goals reached, rewards for accomplishments, what and who you are grateful for on your journey.
8. Relapse Prevention Journal - record of triggers, dates, actions, contingency plan.
9. Relapse Emergency Kit- accountability partner, sponsor and professional emergency contact, in patient relapse rehab options.

Recovery Journaling

Journaling is a beneficial and safe recovery activity. Journaling is a healthy exercise that can improve mental, emotional and physical health and helps with adjustment to life changes and relapse prevention. Journaling can enhance positive affect and optimism. Journaling about past negative events can create positive outcomes as journaling increase self-regulation and self-awareness. Journaling helps a person to spend time in reflection, dig deeper, think about topics on their own and in new ways, and reflect about what has been most meaningful to them. In addition, journaling enhances learning when writing prompts ask reflective questions about participant's learning progress. Journaling is an inexpensive and easily disseminated activity with a favorable risk- benefit ratio.

Chapter 13

Rehab Medications and Dietary Supplements

Currently, there are two medications commonly prescribed to heavy drinkers, naltrexone and acamprosate. These drugs are effective in about 10-12% of people. Programs like Alcoholics Anonymous are more useful than medication, and together outcomes are better than without the other. Many people without sufficient post-rehab support will not quit and stay sober in the long run. There are several, non-addictive substances that may help while you experience the uncomfortable symptoms of rehab, detox and withdrawal for the prevention of relapse through the various stages of your recovery. While the substances are not a cure-all, they have been scientifically proven to be effective as a valid cessation substances along with counseling, education and relapse prevention programs.

Alcohol Recovery Diet & Dietary Tips

For example, research shows that Magnesium may help with pain of withdrawal, like ketamine as it affects the same receptors but without the risk or added adverse side effects. Magnesium supplementation is one of the safest of dietary supplements in doses less than 350 mg. daily are safe for most adults. For information about building a healthy diet, refer to FDA.gov website. For a list of Magnesium rich foods. Other dietary supplements that help the body recover after alcohol abuse are as follows:

Amino-Acids

Amino-acids are found in most protein rich foods. Throughout history amino-acids have been used for depression and brain chemistry imbalances. The use of amino-acids have been used in medicine since the 1900's as one of physician's main methods of treating brain chemistry imbalances before the rise of anti-depressant and mood disorder medications. Amino-acids continue as an option for those seeking natural methods for brain chemistry balancing. Some foods rich in healthy proteins and amino acids, can help the brain make biochemicals innately responsible for good mental health and wellbeing. Providing the building blocks for the brain to recover from alcohol use. The aromatic amino acids:

- tryptophan,
- tyrosine,
- phenylalanine

These aminos are the biosynthetic precursors for the neurotransmitters:

- serotonin,
- dopamine, and
- norepinephrine.

These are some foods rich in amino-acids that help stimulate neurotransmitter production:

Neurotransmitter: GABA	**Neurotransmitter:** Dopamine	**Neurotransmitter:** Serotonin
Amino Acids: Pre-Cursors: Glutamine, Glutamic Acid &	**Amino Acids:** Tyrosine, Tryptophan, & Phenylalanine	**Amino Acids:** Tryptophan, Tyrosine & Phenylalanine
Pre-Cursor Pathway GABA	Pre-Cursor Pathway L-Dopa -Dopamine	Pre-Cursor Pathway 5-HTP - Melatonin
AA Rich Foods: • Almonds • Beans • Brown Rice • Fermented foods • Sauerkrau • Kimchi • Oranges • Spinach	AA Rich Foods: • Aged cheese • Avocados • Berries • Citrus • Eggs • Fish • Oranges • Grapefruit • Lemons • Limes	AA Rich Foods: • Bananas • Chia seeds • Eggs • Fish • Turkey • Mangos • Kiwi • Walnuts • Flaxseed • Sunflower • Sesame Seeds
Amino Acids: Tryptophan, Tyrosine		

Alcohol affects several neurological pathways and causes significant changes in the brain. Alcohol is an addictive drug. The neurological pathways affected by alcohol consumption are the dopaminergic, serotonergic, gamma amino butyric acid (GABA) and glutamate pathways.

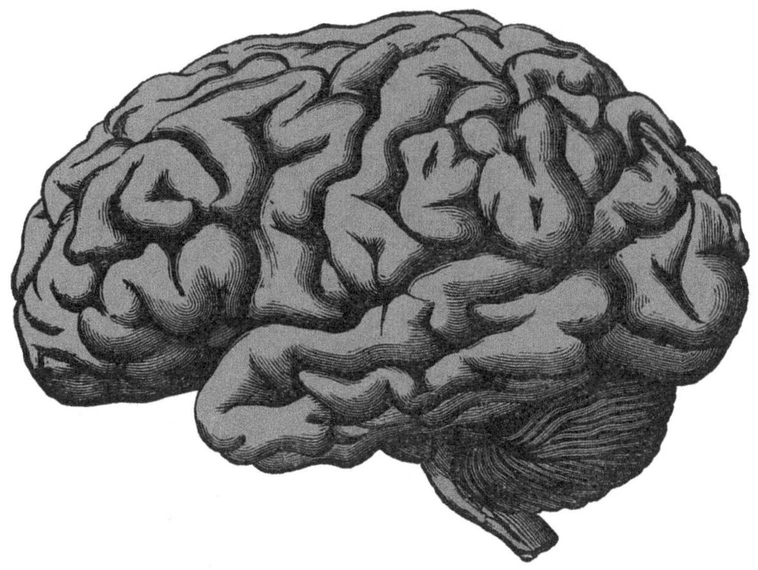

🍸 GABA - Gamma-Aminobutyric Acid

One thing that I found as a helpful solution that helped me after I quit was taking dietary supplements, L-Tryptophan a precursor to the neurotransmitter GABA (Gamma-aminobutyric acid) and both are known as nature's natural valium. Therefore, GABA is only to be taken before sleep. GABA is effective in helping with alcohol cravings and helps lessen pain and withdrawal symptoms. Take Tryptophan, also, at night before bed because if you take GABA during the day, it may make you feel relaxed and sleepy. Alcohol is a depressant and substitutes or mimicks the neurotransmitters on your GABA receptors. GABA deficiency is one of the main causes of withdrawal symptoms and may include:

- depression,
- anxiety,
- insomnia,
- pain,
- slowed thinking
- Decreased mental capacity,
- balance issues and more.

GABA is the brain's most abundant inhibitory, or "calming" neurotransmitter. GABA that is made naturally in the brain has anti-seizure and anti-anxiety effects. Tryptophan is a precursor to GABA and your body can convert into GABA rather than taking a GABA dietary supplement during the day as GABA can make you sleepy. When taken by mouth, GABA is not able to cross the blood brain barrier so eating foods rich in tryptophan can help increase levels of natural GABA. Some Tryptophan rich foods are:

- Turkey/Poultry
- Milk
- Dairy
- Sourcream
- Butter
- Cheese

Tryptophan Vegan Foods:

- Cucumber
- Butternut Squash Seeds
- Soy
- Potatoe
- Walnuts
- Seaweed & Sea Vegetables
- Leafy Greens
- Mushrooms
- Wheat

These are a few natural ways to boost your GABA and Serotonin levels, also. For starters, Certain mind-body practices and exercises may also help boost your brain's levels of GABA. Start taking GABA on the 1st day you stop drinking. Relaxants such as alcohol stimulate GABA receptors, leading to feelings of relaxation and sleepiness. The same effect occurs as a result of taking sleep-inducing drugs. GABA can help with your satiation signals lessening your cravings. An example of an inhibitory neurotransmitter is GABA, which reduces energy levels and calms everything down. Alcohol increase GABA production in the brain, resulting in sedation by increasing the effects of GABA

Produced naturally in the body, GABA is also widely available in supplement form. Manufacturers claim that GABA supplements can help boost the brain GABA levels and, in turn, treat anxiety, stress, depression, and sleep problems. Unlike many dietary supplements, GABA cannot be found in ordinary foods.

When you drink a small amount, you obviously will often only perceive the positive effects of alcohol. But when you drink too much, you can overstimulate GABA pathways, which can lead to extreme sedation of the central nervous system. This can cause alcohol toxicity, blackouts and overdose. Alcohol does the same thing by increasing the effects of GABA. This, by the way, is one reason it is contradictory to drink alcohol while taking Alcohol is a depressant and will cause a person to lose consciousness and pass out into a sleep state. One should never mix alcohol with sleep aids as sedatives such as benzodiazepines as the effects will be amplified, and that can slow the person's heart rate and respiratory system down to dangerously low levels. People have asphyxiated in their sleep by mixing the two drugs.

N-acetyl cysteine (NAC) is another amino-acid that helps abstinence of alcohol consumption for patients with an alcohol use disorder and helps. NAC is an antioxidant with glutamatergic modulating and anti-inflammatory properties. Evidence is emerging that oxidative stress, neuro-inflammation and dysregulation of glutamatergic neurotransmission play a key role in alcohol use disorder. Similarly, oxidative stress is known to contribute to ALD. We outline the studies that have investigated NAC to reduce alcohol consumption including preclinical and clinical studies. We also review the evidence for NAC in other addictions as well as psychiatric and physical comorbidities associated with alcohol use disorders. NAC is a low cost dietary supplement that is well-tolerated by most people and may help improve health after alcohol use disorder in the presence of liver disease.

L Cysteine

Clinical studies have shown L Cysteine, an amino-acid, helps decrease acetaldehyde (a carcinogenic byproduct of alcohol) in saliva and helps in the prevention of digestive tract cancer and breast cancer. L-cysteine supplements offer a variety of health benefits. L-cysteine is available in many foods as well.

- Bean Sprouts
- Broccoli
- Brussels sprout
- Dairy
- Eggs
- Garlic,
- Onions
- Oats,
- Red peppers
- Wheat germ

Cannabidiol (CBD)

We have a natural endocannabinoid system in our body. CBD is found in many plants, but as of to date, in the U.S. the hemp farm bill just became legal but CBD from hemp is still not legal in food products. The great news is, it's not just in cannabis and hemp plants, it is in many other non-restricted foods. In my opinion, CBD is one of the greatest natural medicines ever discovered on the planet! According to the (CDC) Centers Disease Control, CBD is an exogenous cannabinoid that acts on several neurotransmitters involved in addiction. It offers a wide range of therapeutic benefits that may help to alleviate various symptoms and conditions associated with alcoholism. Hemp derived CBD is legal in all states now that president Trump passed the Hemp act and in some states CBD is legal from cannabis, too. However, CBD is found in several other plants and flowers such as moss and echinacea flower stems. In preliminary clinical research on cannabidiol test subjects showed relief of anxiety, cognition, movement disorders, and pain. According to the Research Society on Alcoholism, CBD was found to exert a neuroprotective effect against adverse alcohol consequences, in preclinical studies and CBD appears to have promise as a pharmacotherapy.

Research studies on CBD showed it can effectively reduce addiction relapse provoked by stress, triggers and cues; CBD also reduced anxiety and impulsivity in drug-experienced lab rats. Cannabidiol is a safe and effective natural medicine with many proven health benefits. It can be taken as a vapor, a nasal spray and orally by mouth without the psychoactive tetrahydrocannabinol THC. Additionally, a World Health Organization report states, "In humans, CBD exhibits no effects indicative of any abuse or dependence potential" To date, there is no evidence of public health related problems associated with the use of pure CBD and it is found naturally in many different types of edible plants. Phytocannabinoids have been found to inhibit the breakdown of endocannabinoids and prolong endocannabinoid action. Research has shown that phytocannabinoids offer various benefits.

The U.S. Drug Enforcement Administration Cannabidiol is not scheduled under any United Nations drug control treaties, and in 2018 the World Health Organization recommended that it remain unscheduled.

Phyto-cannabinoids

Phytocannabinoids and CBDs are known to occur in several plant species besides cannabis. Americans and native americans have been using these plants since the founding of the United States, without legal issues and there have been no known adverse side effects. A few of these commonly used plant sources include:

- Echinacea purpurea, Echinacea angustifolia contain CBD.
- Kava plant- yangonin in kava has a positive effect on the CB1 receptors.
- Tea (Camellia sinensis) central nervous cannabinoid receptors may be targeted by some tea catechins, so drink tea when you quit alcohol.
- Limonene gives its plants a lemon smell it is widespread in numerous plants which contain a dietary terpene and beta-caryophyllene identified as a selective agonist of CB_2-receptors. Helps balance symptoms of brain withdrawal.
- Black truffles grow under pecan trees in the U.S. and they contain anandamide. In the healthy brain, cannabinoid receptors are activated by the neurotransmitter anandamide, the "bliss molecule," ananda is the Sanskrit word for "joy, bliss, or happiness." It is likely where these truffles are found growing under pecan trees that pecans contain traces, too.
- Honey - when honey bees feed off the CBD containing flowers from plants containing phytocannabinoids, the honey becomes infused with CBD by nature. Hopefully, these bees aren't labeled criminals for manufacturing CBD infused honey. Often honey contains CBD without anyone ever knowing it is in their

honey. There is a greater honey conspiracy, many of the products labeled honey are not real honey it's syrup. Make sure you are buying real honey.

According to studies, CBD might turn out to be the most effective oral therapy in addiction treatment. Many scientific studies showed positive effects for the treatment of addiction disorders. Although we must respect the FDA's stance and obey the laws regarding CBD. At the present time it is best to stick to the legal food sources of CBD. Study after study, many of them foreign, show the ingredients in hemp-derived CBD as a viable lab-tested pain relief remedy for alcoholism withdrawal symptoms:

- Anxiety
- Nausea
- Chronic pain
- Memory problems
- Diabetes
- PTSD (Post-Traumatic Stress)
- Stress
- Cardiovascular disease
- Several symptoms associated with addiction and withdrawal.

CBD isn't just for those with addiction and medical conditions. In a proper dose, it is safe for everyone suffering with signs of addiction from teens to elderly and it is not only for sick people, its for everyone that wants to improve their health. Healthy people can also benefit from using CBD as part of a preventative health plan. It promotes quality sleep, helps reduce stress and anxiety, and acts as a natural anti-inflammatory agent. There are no scientific studies to date showing any negative side effects of consuming cannabidiol regularly. CBD has actually been extensively studied and proven to have only positive effects. This is part of why it is so appealing.

Self Detox Vrs Medically Assisted Detox

Usually, all light drinkers and most moderate drinkers will be able to quit on their own with this plan. If you are not sure what category your drinking habit falls in, a doctor may determine that and for some moderate drinkers detoxing from alcohol will not be life-threatening or too intensely uncomfortable. Those people are the ones who will be able to self-detox without medical intervention. The other 1-5% will require medical assistance with their detox. The first step is to determine if you qualify for self-detox.

Dietary Supplements

There are some natural and home remedies that help ease mild withdrawal symptoms during the first weeks, still, while the symptoms can get uncomfortable, they are not considered risky.

- Vitamin B1-thiamine. Alcohol use strips thiamine from the body. Over the years, this process can cause Wernicke-Korsakoff syndrome B1-rich foods to the diet can replenish the reserves and relieves mental fog.
- Vitamin C, Selenium, Magnesium, Zinc, and Amino Acids also ease cravings and discomfort.
- Foods like lean proteins offer amino acid precursors to aid the brain in making neurotransmitters
- green vegetables
- Fruit.
- Electrolytes: Drinking water fortified with salts or electrolytes, adding a teaspoon of salt and lemon juice to water, or drinking seltzer water can ease imbalances in sodium and potassium, two very important minerals for mental and physical functioning.
- Melatonin or Valerian for sleep: The natural remedy market has many supplements available to ease insomnia and help a person get a full night's sleep. People experiencing alcohol withdrawal will have a hard time sleeping, so taking small doses of these supplements for a week can ease insomnia and nightmares.
- NSAIDs: Nonsteroidal anti-inflammatory drugs (NSAIDs) like ibuprofen, aspirin ease aches and pains in muscles and joints, relieve mild fevers, lessen headaches and mild symptoms during alcohol withdrawal.

Dietary Supplements- Food, Herbal & Plant Remedies for Rehab

Alcohol is categorised in food and beverages division of the FDA. is plant based with fermented sugar, so it adds a quick burst of energy; when a person stops drinking, adrenal glands may be fatigued from managing these bursts. Herbal remedies can ease this fatigue. Ginseng, rhodiola, or ashwagandha can be found in health stores that supply herbal and vitamin supplements.

DIM- (diindolylmethane)

Alcohol consumption increases your risk of some times of cancers, DIM is a food extract that acts as a hormone balancer and stabilizer in the body. While drinking alcohol increases your risk of cancer, research studies show that DIM may reduce some types of cancers by 30%, including breast, uterine and prostate. DIM is a hormone balancer and stabilizer there are massive amounts of hormone disruptors in various types of alcoholic beverages. Drinking alcohol increases our risk of developing cancer. While DIM doesn't replace medical treatments for cancer, it is an all natural supplement that you can buy over the counter as a daily preventative measure. DIM comes from broccoli but you'd have to eat a ton of broccoli to get the benefits you can get from taking a little 30mg capsule, daily. DIM is not just for women, men benefit from DIM, too. There are so many hidden substances that create a dangerous estrogenic effect in the body, and there are many endocrine disruptors in the environment, everyone could benefit from DIM with no know ill side effects. There are so many other benefits of DIM, too many to mention.

Tryptophan is an amino-acid nutrient found in foods such as turkey and milk. Tryptophan is a natural relaxant. Studies show tryptophan (Trp) helps recovery of alcoholism in 2 ways:

(1) relief of alcohol cravings and recovery from the pharmacological effects of ethanol
(2) improving serotonin manufacturing in the absence of alcohol intake resulting in relief of alcohol withdrawal.

Magnesium- deficiency complicates chronic alcoholism. Magnesium is an essential mineral that is a natural relaxant, however, the body uses up magnesium quickly for many bodily functions, that is why it is also the most deficient nutrient in the American diet. More people are magnesium deficient than any other nutritional deficiency. Magnesium supplementation is generally safe for most people with normal kidney function. Many people eating a normal Western diet have a low intake of magnesium. Those with bowel obstructions, very slow heart rate, or dangerously low blood pressure should not take it. Magnesium can interfere with the absorption of certain medicines such as digoxin, nitrofurantoin, bisphosphonates, and antimalarial drugs. Some food sources of magnesium are whole wheat, spinach and almonds and there is magnesium in mineral water, too.

Alternative Drink Replacements

It is important to have a satisfying drink replacement. Weeks, into my detox, I would still have intense cravings for wine at night so I found a replacement drink to my usual glass of wine. Also, just the habit of years of sipping from a wine glass, at least a few nights per week, when you stop the habit of sipping on something can make you feel like something is missing. My daughter loves Kombucha tea, so I tried it and it was similar to the flavor of my grandpa's wine but it doesn't contain alcohol. I was able to replace wine with Kombucha Tea. I would pour Kombucha in a wine glass for a few weeks, just as a replacement and it worked for me and gave me a sense that I had a replacement that was actually good for my health.

- Kombucha is a fermented black and green tea with fruits and flowers and spices.
- Kombucha starts with a scoby mushroom starter, it is brewed similarly to beer but without alcohol.
- Kombucha comes in many flavors, find the one that satisfies you most.

- Kombucha tastes a little like apple cider vinegar but it's fizzy and refreshing as a light carbonation occurs during the fermenting process but no alcohol forms.
- Kombucha don'ts: there some with small amount of alcohol, those were left to ferment too long, avoid those types at all cost after the first week of your drinking cessation routine.
- Kombucha is beneficial in many ways as it contains probiotics, enzymes and helps rebalance intestinal flora and liver function which was disrupted during alcohol consumption.

The kombucha worked for me! However, kombucha may contain sugar depending on the fruits added so it's not a diet drink by any means. Also, kombucha may be a healthy option for those with certain health conditions, ask your doctor if Kombucha is a good option for you. As for myself, it was a good alternative to wine and it will be good for most as a replacement beverage. If sugar is a problem for your diet, try apple cider vinegar in distilled water as a replacement. Eventually, you can cut back on the Kombucha and even cut it out. Not drinking kombucha containing any alcohol at all is a better option. As the Chinese say 以茶代酒 which means take tea for the replacement of alcohol. Tea can be served hot or cold for many occasions, without harm to your health that alcohol causes.

10 Foods & Drinks That Help You Stay Sober

1. Water- Of course water should be firstly mentioned for alcohol is a diuretic and pushes liquids out of the body. Thus re-hydrating helps people feel better and relieves a hangover headache so it is also important when you quit drinking and all during the rehab phase as alcohol dehydrates the body over a long period of time in chronic drinkers.
2. Tea- Kava, Valerian or Chamomile- according to a PubMed research paper co-authored by Sanjay Gupta on the National Institutes of Health website, titled Chamomile: A herbal medicine of the past with a bright future, it is reported to have positive benefits in the treatment of generalized anxiety disorder and possess suitable effects on seizures. This would indicate that chamomile tea can be of great benefit during detox and rehab as other studies indicate that Chamomile has been reported to help relax nerves, improve sleep quality and aid in the flushing of alcohol from the body.
3. Quit-Aid is a fizzy vitamin and kudzu root tablet that I absolutely love and it's simple, you just drop it into cold or hot water that curbs cravings for alcohol, as it contains extracts, vitamins, minerals and amino acids that help subdue alcohol cravings or a desire to drink alcoholic beverages. It can also be dropped into tea, club soda, tonic water, almond milk, oat milk, cashew milk, rice milk or horchata as it mixes well with any beverage to help control alcohol cravings.
4. Tomato Juice- a liver detoxifier and long used hangover remedy, tomato juice contains glutathione, which the liver uses in detox to help counteract

hangover-inducing toxins, activating the functions of liver to break down and eliminate alcohol but also without alcohol as a virgin bloody mary is a good alternative drink..

4. Celery- is abundant in electrolytes and B Vitamins which alcohol deplete in the body. Celery helps to dispel and replenish the body from the effects of alcohol and relieves upset stomach and flushes out alcohol toxins when drunk. That's why a stalk of celery is also good to include in tomato juice.
5. Eggs- are rich in cysteine and taurine, amino acids that your body uses to produce the antioxidant glutathione which boosts liver function and may help prevent liver disease. Cysteine breaks down acetaldehyde a headache-causing chemical that's left over when the liver breaks down ethanol.
6. Banana- contains potassium and magnesium which alcohol depletes and helps in the process of alcohol excretion. Banana is helpful to ease muscle aches and cramps from electrolyte depletion if a drinker vomits and also helps ease booze blues, therefore, it is a fact that bananas do help ease hangovers and is replenishing.
7. Watermelon- is helpful to offset the dehydrating effects of alcohol which replenishes loss of nutrients depleted by alcohol in the body but also cleanses the body as a diuretic increasing urination and speeds up the excretion of the alcohol metabolite residues.
8. Grapes- are rich tartaric acid and helps turn the ethyl alcohol into ester, weakening the effects of alcohol while easing a queasy stomach. Grapes are the most common type of fruit used in wine-making so eating grapes or drinking small 1 ounce portions of grape juice or sparkling grape juice are non-alcohol forms of wine that can also help decrease cravings for wine.
9. Honey is rich in fructose it can help the body metabolize alcohol more quickly and offset the drop in blood sugar caused by alcohol hangover and help to relieve a hangover headache. CBD honey is from bees who fed off hemp or other plants that contain CBD and it makes a great dual-purpose sweetener.
10. Decaf Coffee- is touted as the best hangover quick fix, still decaf has about 1% caffeine which can help jump start your body through the release of brain chemicals called neurotransmitters. Norepinephrine and epinephrine stimulate several reactions which act as a rescue remedy when the depressant effects of alcohol hangover kicks in. regular coffee has too much caffeine and can complicate a hangover.

Sugar and Rehab

The initial phase of rehab, is far from being a healthy diet. If you go to an AA meeting you will see lots of sweets and sweeteners for coffee and tea. Basically, it is acceptable to use other foods and drinks as a crutch to get off alcohol. In an ideal and perfect world you would only eat a healthy diet, if you can do that while quitting alcohol, you are incredible. If you can't then you can temporarily substitute your alcohol with some of these not so healthy sugar subs and once you have successfully quit alcohol you can work on cleaning up the rest of your diet.

Alcohol Craving Pacifiers

Gum- Chewing gum helps with the flavor cravings there are hundreds of types and flavors of gum you can chew on. Gum can pacify your cravings. There are also medicinal gums. I prefer the natural and neurotropic gum. Just beware of the ones with sugar alcohols commonly found in foods, they are sorbitol, mannitol, xylitol, isomalt and hydrogenated starch hydrolysates. You can't you get drunk off sugar alcohol but it can sure make you sick if you chew too much in a short period of time.

I Overdosed On Gum

Sugar alcohols are not exactly a sugar and they are definitely not an intoxicating form alcohol either. Alcoholic beverages contain ethanol. Sugar alcohols are related to ethanol but do not intoxicate. So you won't get drunk from eating sugar alcohols but just as it did me, it can make you nauseated, vomit and have diarrhea if you chew too much at once. I overdosed on a gum with sorbitol, it was misery. I was sick all night and had a hangover from it the next morning, mostly because it kept me up all night going to the bathroom. You can have up to 3 pieces of gum 3 times a day without the stomach upset or better yet choose one without laxative like artificial sweeteners.

Snack Alternatives

As far as snacking, it is not a good idea to eat the same snacks you use to snack on while drinking alcoholic beverages. If you ate peanuts while drinking beer, it's a good idea to also lay off the peanuts a while as they may be a trigger, for you to drink. I bought snacks that would not pair well with wine, instead of cheese I would eat grapes or apples and veggie snack trays and that helped to curb the cravings and chewing gum helped, too.

Something as simple as fresh fruits, apples and grapes worked well for me, since I was a wine drinker. Pretzels and trail mixes, can be a trigger, so you want to select snacks that you never ate while you were drinking. If you were a martini drinker, then you may not want to choose olives as a rehab snack as those snacks could be a sabotaging trigger. Raw veggies do not typically pair well with wine, so they were a good choice for me and may be a good choice for you, too.

Have a Virgin

If you feel like your missing out have non-alcoholic beer or virgin cocktail. In a class, they look just like their alcohol containing original, just without the alcohol. If your friends keep offering you a drink. You can say, "ok I'm pacing myself on this round I'll have a club soda and lime or go to the bar yourself and order a virgin. You can order most every mixed drink without alcohol and it all looks the same in the glass with a twist of lemon or lime.

The Mocktail: A Mixed Drink Without Alcohol

You can even order an alcohol-free tiki umbrella drink at the beach. If you don't mind the sugar, you can order a juice on ice with a lemon or lime or mint garnish or a glass of tomato juice with a celery stalk or tonic water with a couple of olives, or if you wish you can have a natural grapefruit soda on the rocks and make it a double!

Mocktail Recipes

Delicious Non-Alcoholic Restaurant, Bar & Pub Alternative Drinks:

- Virgin Margarita -soda, lime juice, sweet & sour (frozen or on the rocks)
- Kombucha (hundreds of flavors available)
- Juices on the rocks in a salt rimmed glass
- Sparkling Cider with frozen grapes (in a wine glass)
- Mock Mojito with muddled mint & lime
- Coconut water on the rocks with lime slices.
- Shirley Temple with cherries
- Ginger Ale and bitters
- Cranberry, twist of lime and soda (in a martini glass)
- Non-alcoholic beer, root beer or ginger beer
- Club soda with a twist of lemon or lime
- Tonic water with olives
- Virgin Bloody Mary with Celery Stalk & Olives
- Limeade with a salt rim and sliced lime (in a margarita glass)
- Pineapple juice on the rocks with tiki umbrella
- Sparkling Grape Juice (in a champagne flute)
- A Natural Cola (and make it a double on the rocks).

Homeopathic, Herbal, Nutritional Supplements and Natural Medicines

There are some natural medicines and relaxants that are non-addicting that you may be able to substitute, with your doctors permission, of course, because you should always consult your own personal doctor that helps you manage your health to make sure they approve and that it complements your treatment plan. Some herbs and supplements can interfere with other medications.

Amino Acid Therapy

NAC (N-Acetyl Cysteine) helps neutralize toxins in the liver and boost glutathione levels, while Vitamin C & B Complex supports the body's natural protective enzymes to help you stay sharper and more energetic

DMG (Dimethylglycine) is an amino acid used for the prevention of cancer, alcoholism, and drug addiction that works best integratively along with a rehab and sobriety lifestyle. It is also used for attention deficit-hyperactivity disorder (ADHD), epilepsy, chronic fatigue syndrome (CFS), allergies, respiratory disorders, pain and swelling (inflammation). It is also used to improve speech and behavior in autism, nervous system function, liver function and to improve the body's use of oxygen and to enhance athletic performance. Some people use it to reduce stress and the effects of aging as it also helps lower blood cholesterol and triglycerides and to help bring blood pressure and blood sugar back into normal range. However, it is not a replacement to medication.

Free Form Amino Acids-

Electrolytes alcohol depletes the body, drinking electrolytes replenish lost nutrients and provide hydration to promote healthy muscular and nervous system function

Chemistry Balancer Alcohol wreaks havoc on all bodily systems, alcohol is dehydrating and acidifying in the body the more quickly you can bring your body chemistry back into biochemical homeostasis the more quickly your brain and body will begin to repair and restore itself, after all the body is for the most part, self-healing when it is in a state of homeostasis.

Homeopathic Medicines:

Syphilinum is a homeopathic formula that may help diminish the predisposition to alcoholism in some individuals, while the remedy Sulphur can reduce alcohol cravings in others. Diluting 10 drops of wine, beer or alcohol in a gallon of distilled water and shaking it or sussicating it makes a weak homeopathic tincture. Secretagogues and flower remedies are also helpful homeopathic medicines.

Herbal Medicine:

These are the natural plants that are usually safe, effective and affordable for most people. Ask your doctor prior to taking these and if approved take as directed on the manufacturer's product label or as directed by your doctor.

Valerian Root - Calming and relaxing natural sedative and tranquilizer that is also an anti-convulsant that improves mental function and coordination can offset some alcohol withdrawal symptoms. Valerian comes in capsules, pills, liquid extract tincture or as an herbal tea is helpful reducing for anxiety related to alcohol withdrawal and at bedtime for restful sleep but since valerian antagonises the effects of alcohol and both alcohol and valerian cause drowsiness, they should never be used together. It has been used safely worldwide since the 18th century, it is non-addictive and doesn't make you feel drugged or hung over.

Kava Kava- safe, effective, natural, non-addictive relief for anxiety as a nerve calming plant. However, do check with your doctor first, and do not take if you have hepatitis. Additionally, first check to see if it is legal in your country. It is non-psychoactive and It is my opinion that kava is one of the best natural medicines on the planet for nerves, stress, withdrawal, physical and emotional pain and did I mention, it is non-addictive. Tribal leaders have long drank kava before peace negotiations just as the native people smoked the peace pipe before tribal negotiations, our ancestors used it because they knew it worked to settle agitated people down. As far as speculated liver damage, researchers believe that the liver toxicity comes from kava often being taken with alcohol and that the liver damage is due to alcohol. Never take kava while drinking alcohol.

Passiflora- is a mild nervine and may help improve serotonin levels after alcohol use and helps reduce nervous tachycardia and provides a peaceful easy feeling - benefits insomnia, anxiety, adjustment disorder, attention deficit-hyperactivity disorder (ADHD), pain, fibromyalgia and relieves alcohol and opioid withdrawal symptoms, reducing anxiety and nervousness and reducing heart stress. It contains many compounds that may help restore normal neurotransmitter production, after alcohol dependance.

Chamomile - relaxing calmative tea research shows helps prevent seizures and anxiety which may help with the symptoms of alcohol withdrawal.

Lavender - relaxation essential oil, Lavender oil is one of the best choices for use in aromatherapy to manage the anxiety and psychological stresses related to recovering from alcoholism. According to multiple scientific studies, lavender tea helps calm brain function by triggering chemical reactions in the nervous system.

Prickly Pear Extract helps support the body's natural metabolic response while Milk Thistle promotes liver detoxification activity

Kudzu A widely cultivated herb that has been used in Chinese medicine to control alcohol cravings for over 600 years grows rampantly in the southern United States. Please, do not use poison to kill kudzu, use vinegar or get a few goats and if you have kudzu and have never sprayed it with herbside you can sell it to manufacturers to make into food and herbal medicines.

Angelica Root

Angelica is a potent hepatoprotective herb which will enhance the processes that helps your body expel toxins

Dandelion

Dandelion contains vitamins and nutrients that are crucial to maintain liver health, and increase our bodies ability to detox

Artichoke

Artichoke has been shown to increase bile production which is responsible for enhancing digestion and the absorption of nutrients

Milk Thistle This potent liver tonic has been clinically shown to regenerate the liver, to ensure maximum detoxification efficiency.

Terpenes- have a calming effect and may help lessen the desire for alcohol and offer so many more health benefits. Terpenes are what give some plants a lemon-like fragrance. It is also the compound that drug dogs sniff out in marijuana. Frankincense for example, is high in monoterpenes.

Essential Oils - aromatherapy and aromatic oils have been used to treat minor ailments since the beginning of time. The bible speaks of anointing with oil with implications of healing, mission, sanctification, and exaltation, which bring joy. There are oils and plant compounds that help relieve the signs and symptoms of alcohol withdrawal. Keep a 100% organic essential oil set in your home for personal care, including

- Hemp Oil
- Rosemary,
- Oregano,

- Eucalyptus,
- Tea Tree,
- Clary Sage and more.

Choose oil that is 100% pure organic and laboratory tested for safety. A multitude of uses, from stress reduction to topical first aid.

Epsom Salts/ Magnesium added to warm bath water to topically relax aches and pains of alcohol withdrawal

Thalassotherapy - water is very soothing to the aches of pains withdrawal pains. Detox body scrub, skin brushing and tub soaks with healing essential oils and magnesium bath salts can help make withdrawal more comfortable.

many topical water based therapies comes from the Greek word thalassa, meaning "sea" and is the use of seawater, sea products, and fluctuating temperatures based on shore climate. and body treatments aid in easing the body aches and pains of withdrawal. Soak your body in warm water, Jet Shower, WhirlPool, Jacuzzi - Hot Tub soaks, skin brushing all with sea salts or plant extracts.

Healthy Lifestyle- Adopting a healthier lifestyle can help in the prevention of relapse. In your sobriety add more:

- Organic Foods,
- Clean Air,
- Pure Water,
- Exercise
- Healing Sunshine.
- Nutritional Support

A healthy lifestyle, healthier relationships, healthier mental health, healthy spiritual health and a healthy relationship with self. Detoxify your life, body and mind. Also, energy work is a great therapy. I have released aberrant energy cyst through therapies such as craniosacral therapy. I have released emotional traumas, psychosomatic illnesses through various types of therapy, including massage, adjustments, physical therapy and somatic bodywork.

Mind Body Exercises & Alcoholism- Mind and Body Exercises are proven to increase and regulate serotonin levels, and more studies are being conducted frequently to support the same for dopamine levels. Alcohol causes a decline in these neurotransmitters.

Prayer- Meditation and prayer is very healing. Studies prove there is miraculous power in prayer. If you have faith and believe your prayers will be answered you can expect supernatural help in overcoming alcohol use. I gave up a couple of bad habits through prayer and I have manifested a few great accomplishments through meditation. An example prayer:

> *Dear God, please relieve my pain, take this alcohol addiction from me, forgive me for poisoning my body with unhealthy substances, help me manage my emotions and care for my body as a temple of god as you intended, take all bad habits away and give me the strength to abstain from harmful substances for the rest of my life. Thank you Lord. Amen*

By utilizing prayer, positive thinking and mind body meditations, a person may reprogram their brain to see their life, situations, history, background and relationships in a more positive way. The practice of visual imagery can help you see your life in optimum state, helps dissolve and release painful old experiences. This practice is especially helpful for recovery from childhood emotional wounds. Words are powerful, think up a phrase or mantra that helps you heal your specific hurts and release and let them go, forever. Say the phrase over and over to let go of old baggage, resentment and negative energy that is holding you back in life:

> *"Cup your hand over your own heart. Connect with your own inner pain. Tell yourself. I love you. I am sorry. Please forgive me. Thank you."*

> *Feel the love and joy flood your body like yellow healing sunshine flooding away all darkness, pain and sorrow. Think of something that makes you feel like a child again, something that makes you feel happy inside. For example, if you are an animal lover, think of your pet, a fluffy puppy of kitten. Fill your whole body, mind and spirit with love. Next think of your perfectly happy life. No matter what you don't have, you have imagination. Imagine your happiest life now.*

Several years ago, I became a personal fitness trainer and I designed an Integrative exercise program of 3 Mind-Body exercises that tighten and tone every major muscle group in the body in 15 minutes up to 3 times a day. These, exercises incorporate deep breathing which is important in stress relief. After I finished the Clinical Applications of Mind Body Medicine at Harvard I incorporated breathing exercises into the 3 exercises, to compliment my Mind Body Weight Loss Program book that I wrote years ago when working with my long time friends Amrik and Shami Walia at their Mind Body Center for medicine, where I trained in the Deepak Chopra creating health program, in the late 90's. They encouraged and supported me to incorporate the principles of Ayurvedic medicine into my Mind-Body health programs. I wrote the Mind-Body Type Diet and the Mind Body Exercise Plan, both are of great use, today. It is an anti-aging exercise plan of short burst high intensity exercises, I named "the mind-body exercise program, you can download them on google aps, now, or buy the book is being republished, soon. The Mind Body Exercise program incorporates deep breathing techniques that are excellent for easing stress and anxiety that is associated with all forms of stressful situations, including withdrawal symptoms and exercise compliments any rehab or addiction recovery program because exercise stimulates the feel good hormones that alcohol depletes. You don't need a fancy, gym or expensive workout. You can do them anywhere at anytime in 15-30 minutes a day.

Brain Benefits of Exercise- Exercise causes your body to make feel good hormones, like dopamine and serotonin, this is an important incentive to exercise in addiction recovery. Making a habit of a pattern of physical movement can help prevent a return to alcohol or drug use. Regular exercise done at mild intensity fires up your metabolism, all is needed is enough to make you break a sweat. Sweating is the signal that its enough to get the hypothalamus working and it is a great, non-medical method for treating depression. Exercise raises the levels of the neurotransmitter endorphins, which positively affect your mood. Physical activity also improves sleep and a good night of sleep gives your brain time to repair and recharge neurotransmitters. Many studies indicate that regular exercise can increase alcohol abstinence by 95 percent. These studies also found that exercise can help manage stress, depression and anxiety. This is a good way to lower symptoms of stress and anxiety that may be trigger substance use. Try my mind-body exercise program book its 3 mind-body exercises that tone every major muscle group in 20-30 minutes a day and you can do them anywhere.

Exercise Helps Brain Chemistry After Alcohol- Research shows that vigorous exercises increase levels of neurotransmitters, in particular glutamate and gamma-aminobutyric acid (GABA) which decline with alcohol use and are responsible for chemical messaging between neurons within the human brain. Additionally, endorphins are feel good hormones that is one of many neurotransmitters released when you exercise. Other various physical activities also stimulate the release of brain chemicals, such as dopamine, norepinephrine and serotonin. All of them play an important part in regulating your mood. Vigorous exercise increases neurotransmitters and can help minimize depression and alcohol withdrawal.

Brain Rehab Therapies

Some brain recovery therapies have shown clinically promising results in the ability to better self-regulate drinking behaviors and help to prevent relapse in sobriety. For example, according to peer review studies published by the National Institutes of Health, in a report titled Transcranial Magnetic Stimulation and Deep Brain Stimulation in the treatment of alcohol dependence, the researchers conclude that as of to date, pharmacological and cognitive behavioral treatments for alcohol dependence have achieved limited success. Alternatively, there are some brain rehab therapies that may help those drinkers with liver damage, hepatitis or cirrhosis and that are too sensitive for pharmacological treatments, especially liver transplant candidates and in those cases where effective cognitive behavioral treatments are most needed and abstinence is mandatory to avoid transplant rejection. The following alternatives are promising:

- Transcranial magnetic stimulation (rTMS)is a noninvasive form of brain stimulation in which a changing magnetic field is used to cause an electric current at a specific area of the brain rTMS has shown moderate success, even though it has limited ability to reach several of the key elements in the brain circuit affected by alcohol addiction.
- Mind-Body Medicine techniques are helpful in the treatment of alcohol withdrawal, early-phase detection of clinically promising results in the ability to better self-regulate drinking behaviors. some of the most effective are known as BioFeedBack Therapies. Some examples are:
  Neurofeedback Therapy (NFT) EEQ therapy, also known as "neurofeedback," is a subset of biofeedback therapy that attempts to calm overexcited brain activity.

Mindfulness Meditation	An exercise focused on releasing negative emotions and thoughts through peaceful concentration.
Progressive Muscle Relaxation	An exercise in which recovering alcoholics focus on releasing tension in over-tight muscles in the body, one muscle group at a time by mentally focusing and physically relaxing the tense areas.
Guided Imagery	An exercise directing thoughts toward soothing, positive images and scenarios to relax the mind and body. Using mind over matter. Mind over body.

Chapter 14

Slips and Relapse Risk and Prevention

Relapse means that a former drinker has returned to drinking. A slip is when an ex-drinker is triggered and succumbs to the temptation and drinks a drink before quitting and resuming sobriety. Relapse happens, in part, because of the chronic nature of the disease of alcohol addiction. According to the National Institute on Alcohol Abuse and Alcoholism, evidence shows that roughly 90% of people with alcoholism relapse within 4 years of sobriety. A slip, also known as a lapse, is when someone has a very brief "slip" where they drink, but they stop quickly afterward, avoiding a full relapse into addiction. Others allow a slip to turn into a full-blown relapse or even a total downward spiral until they hit rock bottom or die.

Relapse statistics show that up to 90% of alcoholics will have at least one relapse even after rehab. The percentage of recovery for alcoholics is generally low and alcoholism relapse is high. According to the National Institute on Alcohol Abuse and Alcoholism, up to 90% of alcoholics will have at least one relapse during the first four years after they get sober. However, the way a recovering alcoholic handles a relapse is key to their long-term sobriety. Recent studies indicate that completing an alcohol treatment and rehabilitation program increases your chances of not only avoiding a relapse, but also minimizing the negative effects of a relapse.

Know Your Triggers & Avoid Your Triggers

Staying alcohol-free is a constant battle for recovering alcohol addicts, especially when they find themselves in alcohol-related settings or experience stress or anxiety, which can be a trigger to drink. Without replacement options, the percentage of recovery for alcoholics is generally low and alcoholism relapse is high. The most important things to ensure sobriety success is:

1. Make sure you stay mentally motivated to stay sober.
2. Secondly, take the GABA, nightly, and other supplements mentioned in this book, if your doctor approves, as they may help reduce cravings and help your body resume normal functions and will help to lessen withdrawal symptoms.
3. 3rd, Avoid triggers but don't avoid life, deal with it.
4. Don't Quit on your Quit Drinking Alcohol Cessation plan.

5. Develop Stick-to-it-tiveness.(President Trump, once told me to develop stick-to-it-tiveness, once. He gives good business advice. The main thing I admire about him is that he doesn't drink alcohol)
6. Remember, the death rate of overdose increases with relapse.
7. Get Help- relapse is a sign that you need professional rehab help.
8. If someone is a trigger, take a sabbatical from that person

The Pavlov's Dogs effect, is real and it applies to humans too, especially for alcohol drinkers. Just like Pavlov's dogs were conditioned to salivate when the dinner bell rang, with the expectation of receiving food, the dogs would start salivating; it was a trigger for them to eat. An alcohol drinker's mind and taste buds will start craving a drink when they are triggered, too. Ad campaigns are everywhere, happy-hours are everywhere, it's 5:00 somewhere, a person, a situation, an event such as a ballgame, an anniversary or deceased loved one's death day all of these instances and other stressors can trigger a desire to drink.

Triggers

Triggers are usually memories associated with prior addictive behaviors. The trigger for a recovering alcoholic could be a person, place, thing, or emotion. It could be a person they interacted with in the past or a place they spent time when they were drinking. An emotional situation or stress at work can prompt a return to alcoholism. Alcohol abusers must develop coping skills for these common drinking triggers:

- Happy hour hang outs
- Stressful situations (ongoing marital disagreements, work problems)
- People (bar tenders, drinking buddies, family members, people who are current alcohol abusers, ex-boyfriend or girlfriend)
- Places (bars, neighborhoods, childhood home)
- Smells & Sights (alcohol, seeing others drinking and the alcohol bottles)
- Moods (anger, guilt, loneliness, frustration, depression, fatigue)
- Dates (holidays, anniversaries, birthdays)
- Events (concerts, ball games, reunions)

Recovering alcoholics should avoid these triggers as much as possible while still remaining socially active. Learning to identify triggers, managing cravings until they pass and abstaining without slipping is a crucial component of relapse prevention.

My Personal Triggers

When I go to certain places, it is still a trigger for me. If I go to certain vacation spots where in the past, I would wine and dine or enjoy a champagne toast at sunset. I had to reset my idea of success, it is not about going through life popping champagne corks. Sunsets and a view of the water used to be a trigger for me. Quaint little seaside villages. Waterfront wine bars or restaurants and pretty much all the best places in the world where you enjoy good food and wine by the sea. It is hard to be stronger than your triggers but you can do it. It is hard to order a glass of iced tea when you really want a glass of wine. But once you start drinking your non-alcoholic beverage the craving subsides, it only takes a few seconds to pass on the impulse. No matter where you go on vacation you are likely to be triggered. Enjoy the things that don't involve alcohol and then it becomes easy. It is always 5:00 somewhere and that is where you will be triggered so have your relapse prevention plan in place at all times.

It's always 5:00 somewhere...

Chapter 15

Relapse Prevention Tips

According to research, in the Yale Journal of Biology and Medicine and the National Institutes of Medicine, there are four main ideas in relapse prevention. First, relapse is a gradual process with distinct stages. The goal of treatment is to help individuals recognize the early stages, in which the chances of success are greatest. Second, recovery is a process of personal growth with developmental milestones. Each stage of recovery has its own risks of relapse. Third, the main tools of relapse prevention are cognitive therapy and mind-body relaxation, which are used to develop healthy coping skills. Fourth, most relapses can be explained in terms of a few basic rules. Educating clients in these rules can help them focus on what is important:

1) change your life - to a sobriety lifestyle- don't make it a big ordeal
2) recovery involves creating a new life where it is easier to not drink
3) be completely honest with those you keep company with
4) ask for help - my family would bring me gifts of gum and tea
5) practice self-care and keep your replacement alternatives in hand
6) don't break or bend the rules - walk on past the wine tasting or bar
7) Use Mind Body therapies and wellness care.
8) Talk to a professional counselor or coach.

Remember, to utilize the natural things listed in this book, they can help. An important issue in successful sobriety is the level of alcohol dependence and withdrawal will largely determine the risk of Relapse. An alcoholic often relapses due to a variety of factors including: stress, emotional triggers, inadequate treatment or follow-up, cravings for alcohol that are difficult to control, failure by the alcoholic to follow treatment instructions, failure to change lifestyle, use of other mood altering drugs, and other untreated mental or physical illnesses. Relapses are not always a return to constant drinking and may only be a one time occurrence. However, don't beat yourself up if you slip on an impulse and find yourself having a drink, don't drink the whole thing, throw it away, and remember if you overdose, alcohol poisoning can kill you, alcohol poisoning is no joke. When one quits drinking their tolerance goes down by the day and if they are sober for two months then drink a 5th of tequila they can die and they no longer have the same tolerance as they built up to before quitting drinking. Relapses can be serious and must be dealt with and seen as a high-risk sign to enroll inpatient rehab treatment and recovery. Relapse is a sign that you need professional help. Relapse prevention is an area in the treatment field that is receiving increased attention. Relapse prevention is s basic part of all effective treatment programs. A recovering drinker will need effective relapse prevention activities.

Staying Clean After Detox

The important thing to remember is that for most it is possible to recover from a single slip. Everyone needs an effective, comprehensive relapse prevention plan and worksheet at their fingertips. A good relapse prevention plan outline includes:

- A list of recovery behaviors and plans
- A list of high-risk situations that act as triggers
- Strategies to avoid and escape the trigger situation without relapsing
- Recognize warning signs of impending relapse and prevention

An effective relapse prevention plan will help you develop relapse prevention skills and recovery behaviors which should be practiced on a daily basis before any sign of trouble:

- Maintain a healthy sleeping schedule
- Eat regular meals
- Exercise regularly
- Practice self-care activities, grooming and hygiene
- Practice deep breathing, such as prayana or Holotropic breathwork prove beneficial as a relapse prevention strategy

Bodywork

Studies show that physical healing modalities are associated with positive changes in the endorphin system, wellness therapies such as Osteopathic Manipulation Therapy, Massage Therapy, Chiropractic Adjustments, Physical Therapy, Cranio-Sacral Therapy, Spinal Alignment Technique, Acupressure, Acupuncture, Whirlpool contrast therapy and more, may actually be mediated by the endocannabinoid system which can help with withdrawal type symptoms, alcoholism and addiction. Additionally, touch therapies have been shown to increase hemoglobin and therefore must stimulate other healing mechanisms in the body that are beneficial for a sense of well being.

Alcohol Induced Brain Damage

One of the side effects of alcohol abuse is brain damage and injury. It has been cited in many research papers that alcohol robs the body of man nutrients and can cause thiamine deficiency which can result in brain injury. However, alcohol has a number of other damaging effects on the brain, including:

- Depletion of amino acids and nutrients that are needed by the brain glands and tissues to manufacture neurotransmitters
- Direct organ damage, injury or death of brain cells including neurotransmitters and their receptors and receptor sites
- Alterations in brain chemistry and brain chemicals including neuropeptides, neurotransmitters or the manufacturing of the hormones the brain produces to regulate the function of every organ & body system.
- Oxygen deprivation to brain tissue and brain cell death

Alcohol Induced Deficiency And Wernicke-Korsakoff Syndrome

Alcohol abuse can result in brain damage by interfering in the absorption, assimilation and utilization of the nutrients required to maintain good brain health and organ function. Alcohol causes a myriad of brain chemistry imbalances. An example of this is Korsakoff's Syndrome, which is a result of thiamine deficiency. Wernicke's encephalopathy and Korsakoff's psychosis are two of the more commonly known conditions caused by alcoholism. Wernicke-Korsakoff syndrome is one name for both conditions because they often happen together.

Thiamine Deficiency Symptoms:

- Loss of Appetite
- Fatigue
- Irritability
- Agitation
- Frustration
- Slow Reflexes
- Nerve Damage (Tingling Arms and Legs and Nerve Pain)
- Muscle Weakness
- Blurry Vision
- Nausea or Vomiting

Thiamine, is vitamin B1 and it has a ph stability point of 5.0-7.5 and because alcohol is a weak acidic with a pH below 5 alcohol depletes B1 from the body of Thiamine overtime as it is not able to be produced by the body, which means it must be ingested through foods containing thiamine because it is required by nearly all the tissues in the body, including the liver, heart, and brain. However, alcohol interferes with the body's ability to absorb thiamine, resulting in deficiency. Some foods rich in thiamine are:

- Seafood
- Lean meats
- Poultry

- Eggs
- Legumes (beans and peas),
- Nuts
- Seeds
- Soy

Brain Rehab Therapy

Breathwork Pranayama originates from Ayurvedic medicine and is the formal practice of controlling your breath, which is the source of our prana which is a person's vital life force. Mindful breathing is also a Mind Body exercise that helps lower stress, pain and anxiety and helps with withdrawal symptoms. Breathwork, works, you can get an oxygen high and it helps to skip the urge to drink.

High-Risk Trigger Situations

It is a good idea to make a relapse prevention plan ahead of time. Certain situations specific to each individual can put a person who is abstaining from drinking, at risk of relapsing into drinking again, these situations are called "triggers" and they are known to cause slips and relapses:

- Strong emotions- anger, worry, grief
- Change, different schedules at home/school/work
- Health challenges- withdrawal pain
- Stressful marital, family or social issues
- Loss of a loved one, pet or a death in the family

Early trigger warning signs

Triggers should be recognized and addressed early to prevent a relapse:

- Emotional detachment
- Skipping work
- Neglecting health
- Depression

Your relapse prevention plan should include strategies to cope with particular situations and get back on track. An effective program has two main components:

- A strong, comprehensive support system of family, friends, and professional caregivers
- A willingness to take action to prevent momentary slips
- A firm commitment and determination not to return to drinking alcohol

Learning about relapse and preventing it with a strong will to quit and deal with setbacks such as slips and relapses. Stay strong. Stay positive. That's the only way to beat alcohol use or addiction and enjoy life to the fullest.

Helpful Relapse Prevention Activities Are:

Guided Imagery and Self-Hypnosis. Envision you're sober living. Get a good clear picture of yourself without alcohol and burn that image in your mind. While you are fully aware of how your life was with alcohol in it, can you envision your life once you have completely stopped drinking. Meditate on your sober self, daily.

- Visualize yourself as a stronger, sober, happy and healthy person, where you will be in a day, week, month or even year.
- Imagine your new self and look into the future, see how it is better without booze this will provide you with inspiration
- Do the shadow work, that is needed to work through the root cause of your alcohol abuse problem
- Know you can achieve your overall goal of sober living.
- Know it is not going to be as hard as it is today forever. It gets easier.
- Get therapy if necessary - addiction counseling, psychotherapy, hypnotherapy, equine therapy, cranio-sacral therapy, mind-body medicine, pharmacotherapy, therapeutic massage and chiropractic.
- Take up a class- painting, sculpting, wood work, arts & crafts
- Creative outlet- learn a new skill - music, song writing, poetry
- Avoid situations in which you drank alcohol before sobriety
- Avoid places where you drank before sobriety
- Go to a sobriety group meeting or an encouraging counselor
- Have an emergency accountability partner 24/7
- Have other substitute drinks and mocktails readily available
- Take up a new healthy hobby, join a meetup group
- Join a church - support group, pray, work on spiritual self.

Other People Sabotagers Of Sobriety

You may even have to avoid people who side-rail your sobriety, people who may intentionally trigger your stress. Tell people whom you previously drank alcohol with that you are sober, take a sabbatical from them if they are not willing to respect, support, encourage and celebrate your sobriety.

Society Expectations

Recovery is something you do for the rest of your life. Enjoy live be present for every moment of it. If you are struggling with alcohol, get the crap out of your body and start to live again. You will be surprised people want to help you if you want to help yourself.

Sobriety Tempting People

You may be surprised to discover, some people don't want you to become sober. You may be even more surprised when people who nagged on you about your drinking will attempt to temp you. Also, those who expressed they wanted you to quit for years may start tempting or triggering you during your detox or some point in early sobriety. They will doubt you and your sobriety and test it. They may go so far as to temp you intentionally, to see for themselves, before they will believe you are sober. They will be amazed by your sobriety and find it unbelievable that you have gone stone-cold sober. They will want to temp you to see if you are really sober, so, beware! Those are the people who will test you and temp you with a "set-up". It starts out with them plotting up a "set-up" to test you. These people are sometimes are the people you would least expect, usually friends or family members that may not even drink themself. Do not meet with these tempters or tempstresses at the time of day that you may experience anhedonia as they may push our will power over the edge.

The sobriety tempter or temptress will:

- Offer to buy you a drink, after you've already told them you've quit.
- Bring you a bottle of champagne to celebrate something.
- Press you to go to a bar when your suppose to go to dinner.
- Choose a mexican restaurant when they know tequila is your trigger
- Call and tell you they are in wine country and the vineyards are beautiful
- Call at when they are at a happy hour and ask what your doing
- Call you from a cruise where they are playing drunk limbo
- Bring up upsetting situations from the past to trigger your nerves

Sobriety Tester

These are people who know you really well. They know you better than anyone knows you. They are your sober friends or family members, a sibling, they know things about you that other people don't. They know your weaknesses. They know your heartaches, past betrayals and they know your fears. Learn to look for the signs this before the set-up happens to you because it could cost you your sobriety by causing you to slip or relapse and fall out of sobriety.

The "Sobriety-Tester"

- Will intentionally trigger you by pushing your buttons to test you to see if you'll drink during or after their stress creating encounter.
- They stage a "set-up" by cornering you and starting a confrontation or
- Start a passive conversation about something that they know will push your buttons and upset you.
- The "sobriety-tester" will intentionally trigger you by bringing up past hurts to see if you'll drink during or after their stress creating encounter.

Some of these sobriety testers want you to continue drinking for their own selfish reasons. They are corruptors. They are destroyers. They are evil in my opinion. How dare they to try to sabotage your struggle to sobriety. How dare they to temp you. These are what I call the sobriety werewolves, they are waiting to attack your sobriety for various selfish reasons and they will go in for the kill of your sobriety. Why would someone do that, if they love or care for you? If you are getting together with people for the first few times of your sobriety, be prepared to be "set-up" and tested.

Examples "Set-Up" Triggers Sobriety Testers Will Use

- They will bring up a past betrayal and pick at every detail to upset you
- They will bring up a business deal that fell through that use to upset you
- They will bring up an unresolved family issue just to trigger you about it
- They will bring up the family trouble maker to gossip with you about it
- They will bring up all the things that they know upset you in the past
- They will deliberately overwhelm and pester you
- They will trigger the problems that you drowned with alcohol in past
- They will bring up an ex who did you wrong
- They will ruminate your past emotional injuries

Sometimes, the people you love the most will test your sobriety. It may be ex's, manipulating partners, family members, friends or lovers will fear your sobriety. It is usually the people who had some control over you or maybe someone you allowed to control you when you were a drinker. Some will feel threatened by your sobriety that somehow, they won't be able to control you or fear that you won't need them in your life anymore or fear that once your clean, they will have to clean up their act, also. They may fear they cannot manipulate you to do what they want you to do, once you are sober. You will know who these people are the moment they trap you into a trigger "set-up. They put you in a stressful situation to see if you will drink again.

During a Trigger "set-up" you have choices:

- You can try to explain to them that their actions are triggering you and ask them to stop
- You can explain to them you are in a sensitive withdrawal state and ask them to help you get through it and go have a non-alcoholic beverage, together.
- You can leave the "set-up" and walk away
- You can turn the "set-up" around and call them out
- You can take a sabbatical from having a relationship with them (if they are a drinker or user themselves)
- Recognize their intentions & do not be tempted nor triggered to drink! (do not submit to drinking alcohol)
- Do not give anyone the power to trigger you into relapse
- You are in control of your triggers and your sobriety.

Ultimately, you have to be strong to protect your sobriety. You have to protect your sobriety until your strong enough to overcome your personal triggers. You deserve your freedom in sobriety. Don't let anyone rob you of your sobriety. Someone who sabotages your sobriety, does not really care for you or truly love you. Sobriety is your good health and well being. Sobriety is a gift. Sobriety represents your future success in life. Sobriety is a treasure that you need to protect. Sobriety is overcoming the beast. In sobriety, you are a stronger person with more control, you are a winner in life.

Relapse Death Risk

Relapse increases your risk of spiralling out of control into alcoholism and can lead to death. The longer you are sober the lower your tolerance becomes, if you use to drink a ⅕ of vodka, a few weeks into sobriety and you body can only tolerate a few drinks without developing alcohol poisoning and it can be more of a fatal risk, than before. The early stages of your sobriety are fragile and must be handled with care. It is important to reduce the risk of being triggered and reduce exposure to triggers for a significant amount of time. Until you are no longer dependant on alcohol and until you can abstain without feeling an internal impulse or until it is no longer a struggle for you not to drink. Even if you are a strict believer in moderation, alcohol dependence can sneak up on you and so can a relapse. I thought I was the last person in the world that drinking wine could become a habit or problem. I always said I could take it or leave it. I was in denial that wine was alcohol. I did not see wine as being as bad as liquor. Until I came to the realization, and admitted they were the same. Wine is as detrimental as liquor when it is over consumed it is alcohol abuse. Mom was right, people can become a wino. In my denial, I didn't view a wino as being an alcoholic. In my sobriety, I realize that in fact, yes they are both one and the same. I didn't want to admit the truth, that is the essence of denial. Alcohol just like every other addictive drug. If you continually use it you will become dependant. You can overdose on Alcohol.

I Think I'll Drink Myself To Death, Today

Virtually, none of the alcohol drinkers who die from alcohol, woke up that day and said, "I think I'll drink myself to death, today". Usually, deaths come after an alcohol overdose. Alcohol overdose occurs when you drink too much alcohol, too quickly. During early sobriety, past drinkers are especially vulnerable to alcohol poisoning during a relapse or slip. During early sobriety, tolerance to alcohol is decreased while the cravings remain the same it is this combination that can prove fatal during a relapse. The greatest risk to a person who is in early treatment and who relapses is the threat of overdose because they do not have the same alcohol tolerance they previously built up to as a former alcoholic, after a period of sobriety, they have no tolerance but they still have a big craving, they are vulnerable to alcohol overdose during a relapse, they also they often have poor judgment in discerning how much they should be drink during a relapse and usually consume a large quantity that causes alcohol poisoning. Once too much alcohol is used, it enters the brain stem area and it may cause a drinker to lose consciousness, pass out and depresses the nervous system and respiratory center, and you may stop breathing or it may cause the over drinker to vomit causing asphyxiation. That's one way how drinker's die.

When Rehab Is Mandatory

Some of the mental and emotional symptoms that may follow an alcohol relapse can make it difficult for a person to admit to a need for professional treatment, including:

- **Near Death Experience** A drinker that may have survived more than one serious alcohol related poisoning or overdose episode and does not quit.
- **Relationship Problems or Domestic Violence** Angry suppressed emotions taking it out on others. Blaming others for being the problem when your drinking is the problem. Drinking is damaging most of your relationships.
- **Criminal Charge** - drinker has legal problems or DUI arrest
- **Denial** a person who has suffered a great loss due to their drinking and tries to convince themselves that they don't have a drinking problem and that they don't need help to quit drinking
- **Hopeless -** Thinking that treatment won't work because they are too far gone with their drinking.
- **Negative Thinking** They think thoughts such as, "What's the point?
- **Previous Relapse** Treatment obviously didn't work last time or I wouldn't have relapsed."
- **Rehab Adherence** Drinker isn't following their counselors homecare recommendations utilizing learned prevention skills. The skills learned in treatment are still helpful, but a refreshed approach is needed.
- **Making Excuses**. don't have the time or money for therapy.

- **Depression.** If a person berates themselves for their drinking so much that they feel like everything in life is pointless.
- **Suicide** drinker who is thinking of committing suicide is a mandatory time to go to treatment in a supportive environment that can help regain hope and their love for themself and life.
- **Loss** drinking is causing a drinker not to be able to be independant becoming unable to support themselves due to drinking
- **Counseling** drinkers who have relapsed a return to use is not the end of the story. It is possible to build a better life after one or more relapses, every addict needs a good counselor to go to when at risk.

For those who have slipped or relapsed rehab may be important for long term success in sobriety, to occasionally update the alcohol relapse prevention plan on a periodic basis: once a month for the first 3 months of relapse recovery, quarterly for the first 2 years and then on an annual basis, as necessary, thereafter. This is important for previous drinkers who relapse because every stage of recovery has different support needs. What was a trigger for a person 12 months ago may no longer be a trigger, now they may have new triggers.

Sober Living Recovery Houses

Recovery houses are another option that can help newly sober individuals during initial alcohol recovery. They provide a range of free services to individuals in recovery including counseling support, job search, life coaching, sober housing, government resources, recovery workshops, resource links, training, and volunteer networking opportunities. Among other goals, these services aim to facilitate the entry level rehab individuals into a supportive community and to bridge the gap for individuals exiting treatment discharge back into society within their communities.

Governmental Policy Good News

There is hope. There are many new governmental community health programs and counseling methods available that you can utilize that will help you quit drinking and if you have a will to quit there are many ways to help yourself and many options for professional help if you feel you can't quit on your own. The Mental Health Parity and Addictions Equity Act is designed to expand mental health and substance use disorder benefits and federal parity protections for more than 60 million Americans. New health plans are now required to cover preventive services like depression screenings for adults and behavioral assessments for children at no additional cost. And starting next year, insurance companies will no longer be able to deny health care coverage to anyone because of a pre-existing mental health condition. This can open the door for more people to opt into recovery treatment. Additionally, there are many substance abuse counselors. There are many rehab programs available. Our government agencies offer the "Rethinking Your Drinking" campaign and there are more public awareness campaigns in the making. Additionally, recently legislation has been proposed for more funding for better public alcohol safety campaign announcements. All of the aforementioned professionals are available to help if your drinking has gotten out of your control. These professionals are working hard to help educate the public regarding alcohol use and abuse. The National Institutes of Health (NIH) & U.S. Department of Health and Human Services offer a free educational hand book titled "Rethinking Drinking" on their website by the National Institute of Alcohol abuse and Alcoholism. Alcohol awareness campaigns are beneficial to us all since 70% of our population drank alcohol last year. Better programs will help keep ourselves and our communities safer. Studies show communities that limit the times alcohol is sold as something that's been shown to reduce alcohol's risk of causing harm. The lighter the concentration of stores that sell alcohol in a particular area, the less people will drink.

Alcohol use and Divorce & Break-up

According to NIH researchers, compared to their married counterparts, divorced individuals, have higher levels of psychological distress, substance abuse, and depression, as well as, lower levels of overall health. The most common "final straw" reasons for divorce were:

- Infidelity or other form of trust betrayal
- domestic abuse or violence, and
- alcohol and substance use.

However, the research also shows that you're more prone to drinking when you're betrayed or rejected by someone you're much closer with, like a best friend, a family member or a romantic partner.

Rock Bottom

Every drinker will hit their rock bottom at some point, it is different with each person. Usually, people will wait for their rock bottom moment before they give up drinking. Sadly, some will not quit until they get a DUI or have a wreck or other serious life problems. Unfortunately, for some, that rock bottom is a near death experience. Hopefully, you will decide to quit before you almost die. I quit for my health, I quit for a better life, I quit for my daughter because I don't want to put her through any similar pain she suffered because of the circumstances of her father's death. I quit for my mom because she was right, I wasn't an alcoholic but with my drinking behavior I could have potentially become a wino and lastly, because at one point I realized that a healthy glass of wine, was not healthy at all because of a big cover up that was revealed across the media about grape farms where my favorite wine came from was not truly organic grapes the overused fields were tainted with chemical residues of herbicides and pesticides, which are endocrine disruptors and that is one of the major reasons I initially decided to quit. I will not knowingly consume cancer-causing poison. I had an awareness moment that alcohol is a sort of slow poisoning the body without even over drinking. I knew in my heart that I had to quit or die from consuming the inadvertent toxins. Additionally, I realized that many of my clients that were coming to me for beauty and aesthetics, had addiction or alcohol use problems and that I could not be completely healthy and set the best lifestyle example for my clients unless I could live in that example myself. In order to best help them connect to their motivation for recovery with integrity, I had to quit. I quit for myself and my patients because as a healthcare giver, it is important to be authentic. Lastly, those who are supernaturally gifted from God, to be caregivers and those who are christians must believe in and follow the words of Jesus, physician heal thyself first.

Rock Bottom Relapses Into Drinking and Codependency

Everyone has a rock-bottom in their drinking life, if you are one of the lucky ones and you survive it, you will, always remember that point and once you go down that path, you will never go down it again, if you can learn from your mistakes, they can help you stay sober. The following are a couple of stories people shared with me during my research on alcoholism, real people sharing their relapses and what it was like to hit rock bottom, before they quit drinking.

Anonymous Testimonials

Tragic Drinking Stories With Victorious Endings:

Alcohol Recovery Story #1

Hey there Dr. Joy, Just wanted to drop you a note and let you know how I'm doing.. I am doing well and It feels good to be back in control of my life, again after giving up alcohol.. Looking back, before alcohol, I was usually always in control of my life and after my fiance' cheated on me with my best friend, I grew bitter. I didn't realize I was using alcohol as a crutch but in reality, I started drinking heavily after the break-up and my life was a mess for quite a while after that. I shut down and basically became counter-dependant. For a long time, i wouldn't get too close to anyone.. I was a man who pushed everything and everyone out of my life, at the first sign of any drama, Needless to say, life became very lonely and I drank alcohol to numb my physical needs and desires. I gradually became alcohol dependent. The main reason I drank was because I was feeling betrayed and also from being lonely and not having a companion in life that I felt I could trust. I was traumatized and became cold hearted from alcohol. I would break up with a woman the second she became needy in anyway or if anyone caused any stress in my life, I would cut them out, like dead wood. Unfortunately, porn and bourbon became my companion.. Like so many other drinkers, whiskey had me so numbed up emotionally, that I wasn't feeling my real feelings and at times it also affected my making good decisions. I had opportunities to be in a good relationship with a couple of really fine ladies, but I would test them and if they didn't put me first or didn't excite me enough, I cut them out. Still, deep down inside I wanted to share life with someone special and to try to be in love, again. I started talking to a counselor about a year ago and he helped me with my trust issues and suggested that I cut back on my drinking, that's when I found you and started your quit drinking system and detox was hard but three months into this, I still can't believe, I've given up alcohol and I don't feel I need it anymore. I am also in a new relationship with a non-drinker, she's amazing with a natural zest for life. This is a first for me, and I'm feeling happier everyday that goes by without the bozos and the booze.. Thanks Tom R.

Alcohol Recovery Story #2

Dear Dr. Joy, I am a business owner, I never thought I could develop a problem with alcohol, but I was well on my way of doing so before starting your quit drinking program. One night, I was stressed to my max, I couldn't sleep, I was in pain from an auto injury, I was grieving my mother's death. I was alone and I was so upset over a break up and intimate relationship betrayal. I drank too much and got alcohol poisoning, but luckily I survived. A friend that I loved and trusted betrayed me while knowing everything else I was going through, when I needed them most. Everything came to a head in my life, all at once. I was in disbelief that after 25 years of freedom from an abusive alcoholic marriage and divorce, I found myself drinking and worse than that, i was back in another codependent relationship with someone who had a very troubled past, but they were not the drinker, I was. When I first met him, he presented himself as a successful, loving family man type so I gave him a chance to be friends and over time I had grown to love him. He was exceptionally talented in many ways and super intelligent and I could see great potential from the beginning of our relationship but because of our troubled past, I was reluctant to get deeply involved. I insisted we go to family counseling to improve our relationship potential and we went to relationship counseling together. Personally, I thought that because of going to couples classes in the beginning of our relationship that we would have a more solid foundation to build a relationship on, and that we would never put each other in jeopardy by a breach of trust. However, therapy doesn't fix anyone's character flaws unless they want to change. A person generally has a proclivity of being honest and trustworthy or they don't. When I found out that a loan was taken out in my company's name without my knowledge or approval by an acquaintance of his, I felt betrayed that my he would carelessly bring someone who became a danger to my company's reputation and my own livelihood into my circle. The borrower was a business partner of his, the lender was an acquaintance of his which I never met. I felt duped by both, I couldn't imagine that he would get involved with someone who would do that to me behind my back! However, I found out that it wasn't my friends fault and that the lender had forged other peoples loan documents in the past and in fact gone to prison for it. The lender set us both up in an attempt to extort us. My friend took care of paying the loan, but, I made a pact to never trust him again, or be involved with any of his shady business contacts ever again. I was angry to have my trust betrayed in such a detrimental way. I was angry at myself for trusting people that my gut warned me all along not to trust. I didn't realize there are those types of white collar crooks in the world or that they would try to put me in the middle of their bad business deals without my knowledge or cause stress in my life over their private business which I had no involvement in. I started seeing a counselor and decided to clean my life up. I found your quit drinking tablets and attend a weekly support group. I am now off alcohol for 9 months and feeling better thank I have in a long time. Kind Regards, Sandra K.

Story #3

Hi Doc, I love your quit-aid products and I want to share more of my story with you. I was using alcohol to cope with my relationship issues with my boyfriend. It all came to a head when I was in an emotional crisis. I was in disbelief that even after I went to therapy with my boyfriend, he did some secret business deals behind my back and got himself involved with a shady business partner and, he didn't protect us and got himself into a situation that allowed his business partners to potentially cause harm to us. I received court documents from a loan company, my company was being sued for a loan which I did not apply for, turns out my boyfriend took a loan out in my company's name posing himself as an owner in my company, within a month of discovering the betrayal, I lost my trust in the relationship and he claimed he was traumatized, too, that the company had produced fake loan documents. Turns out it was true, one of the loan officers had been charged in the past for forging loan documents. We were both distraught and I was upset that he allowed other people to put us and our livelihood in jeopardy. To make a long story, short, we chose to take time apart and we took a four month sabbatical from each other. I needed time alone and he had work he needed to do to straighten this mess out, he had some other family business out of town, too. I had to face some harsh realities on my own and process the extent of the damage to our relationship. It was a trust betrayal and any self-respecting person will either end the relationship or take time to determine the appropriate actions to repair a relationship and if the relationship is salvageable, the proper steps to take to insure the same mistakes do not ever happen again. I didn't want to cut this person out of my life forever, because I had grown to love him dearly, yet, I wasn't going to be betrayed or taken advantage of or disrespected by his associates either. I drank for a few years to cope with the stress of this relationship and the betrayal but since I finally decided to quit, your system is what helped. I have been sober since New Years Day, 7 months and counting. Quitting has helped me get my life back on track. Thanks for your help, it worked! Thank you. JK

Alcohol Fatal Crutch In Life's Darkest Hour

When people find themselves in a difficult phase in life, many make the mistake of turning to alcohol as a crutch to numb their pain.

Alcohol Recovery Story #4:

I am a bank manager and my job is quite stressful. For a few years, I had made the mistake of using alcohol as an emotional crutch after my divorce. One day I got the news that my ex husband surprised us all and had gotten married to a family acquaintance. I couldn't believe who he was married to, it was someone I did not want to be around my children and I was disappointed in my ex's choice of a step mother for our children. I remember I felt helpless that day the two of them came to pick up the kids for weekend visitation. I opened a large bottle of wine and began drinking. My drinking almost came to an ugly and fatal end on that unsuspecting night. My rock-bottom was a near-death experience. I should have called a friend but chose to self-medicate my pain with alcohol, I wasn't in the mood for company as I still had some thinking and drinking to do over what to do about handling my problems. I was angry at him for being tricked into a whirl-wind relationship and marrying someone that i knew would let him and my children down in the end. I was very disappointed not only in him but in myself as I found myself enabling his bad relationship behaviors and I did not want that person of bad character in my childrens lives. I didn't understand how could this have happened, after getting all the bad relationships out of my life successfully,

I found myself back in another situation with their dad's new wife who was a textbook evil stepmother type that would be a bad influence on my children. I knew she had too many character flaws and shady people around her. It was their turn to have our kids for visitation for the weekend so I took some much needed time to myself, so, I fled the city and went to my country home, alone. As I drank a bottle of wine, I internalized the emotional pain and hurt, and was triggered like a ghost from the past crashing all of my good sense and healthy boundaries down. I chose to drown my sorrows by drinking wine and I didn't stop until the whole bottle was gone. I made the mistake of thinking I could drive a few blocks away and buy some more… wrong! I was pulled over by the police for rolling through a stop sign. I got a D.U.I. it took that to see that I had problem I had to deal with, too. It was embarrassing, here I was thinking I was the responsible one but I learned the hard way, that even smart people can make stuipid mistakes when it comes to alcohol misuse. Lesson learned, don't drink and drive and if something is bothering me now I deal with it or talk to a counselor, a friend or a family member. You can't drown problems with alcohol. I quit by using your system, I only wish I would have quit sooner before I ruined my driving record.

Thanks, Ingrid S.

Alcohol Story #6

Hey Doc, When I first went To college, last fall, I almost died from chugging alcohol. i beer bonged a boiler-maker, in case you don't know what that is, its a bottle of whiskey Mixed with beer. It was a bad idea, I woke up in the hospital. Apparently, I almost died from alcohol poisoning. I was so sick and They pumped my stomach and pumped me full of black detox charcoal because I had the stuff all over my face. When I woke up. After I got out of the hospital my parents gave me a gift basket one of the items was your quit-aid, it helps me not to want to drink so much and i will never do anything crazy like that with hard alcohol again. I rarely ever drink now but when I do Go out to have a drink with friends, I drink the quit-Aid first and only have a beer or two at most. I quit over drinking and maybe I will quit for good, someday, too. Thanks jay D.

Alcohol Story #7

Dear Dr. Joyce, I use to self-medicate with alcohol. Once, I did what so many drinkers make the mistake of doing when they are stressed and in emotional pain. I decided to drink to numb my hurt and loneliness to put myself out of my misery so I could sleep. Before, I realized, I drank a whole bottle of tequila. I guzzeld 16 shots all in only a few hours. This was a dangerous thing to do. Was in the hot tub to try to relax when the effect hit me in an adverse way, with all the cortisol and adrenaline rushing through my blood, that the tequila made me sick in a way I had never experienced before, in fact, it made me deathly ill. It hit me hard, before I could even realize what was happening. I was blacking out and I could not get out of the bathtub. I was so sick I felt instantly nauseous like I would vomit but I had overdosed and my body was out of my control at that point. I was so weak I couldn't stand up. I was on the verge of passing out, and it was like climbing the hardest mountain to lift my hand and manage to press the lever to turn off the jets and drain the water from my bath to keep from drowning.

Still, after the water was gone, I could not move, I felt I was going to die in my hot tub not from drowning but from alcohol overdose and poisoning, something that at that point I had not even realized it could happen, until it did. I felt paralyzed and I realized I had alcohol poisoning. My heart was racing from the heat and stress hormones. I knew I was at risk of a medical emergency and all I could do was pray for to god to help me, please, don't let me die like this. I asked god to please let me recover that night and I would never over-drink again but if it was my time to go, to please, take me in any other way. I promised I'd never over drink like that again. 911 was out of reach as my phone was upstairs in my bedroom on the battery charger. It took all of my mind-body strength and at least a half-hour just to get out of the tub. I sipped water to try to neutralize the alcohol and purge it out of my body, after urinating I finally was able to drag myself 40 feet away to the kitchen to take an alcohol detox drink and it was my only hope to dilute and flush some of the alcohol out. I'm sure I almost died. After my alcohol poisoning episode was over, I thought about what it would be like dying this way and how painful it was being in that debilitated state, but then I thought about how painful it would be for my family I knew better, I was ashamed for trying to drown my anger, hurt and disappointments in life with tequila instead of dealing with issues. After that night, I saw a counselor and she's helped me develop better coping strategies and then I found you and got on your plan too, your quit drinking products worked, too! This is amazing to me because I don't even want to drink alcohol now, and before, I never thought I would ever quit drinking. I made a vow to myself to make my life better and took action, I quit alcohol, and I know if I can do that, I am strong enough to deal with anything. Now, I am alcohol-free, joined a health club and mostly drink fruit laced water, tea and coffee. I will never touch alcohol again, it's a killer! Thank you. Tina R.

Alcohol Recovery Story #8

Hello Dr J, As you know, I am a musician and I had been a drinker that was getting out of hand. After my overdose, I went to rehab and after I got out I took the steps to detox if i hadn't I likely would have died. It took a drama-king to come into my life like a wrecking-ball, to break down my rebellious walls. He showed me such passion for life, he knocked me and my life off the dangerous course it was on, I found balance again and your program woke something up inside me that had been dead or numb for a long time, from drinking. He set up my first visit with you and within two weeks, it was enough for me to snap out of my addictions. Turns out he was right and I was wrong, I can live without alcohol. Glad he became a tee-totaler before I met him and he showed me the way he didn't drink alcohol anymore. He had a wounded broken past, like me. I found someone that I could heal and grow with. You taught us both how to take our personal power back and I quit drowing my heartache, pain and sorrows with liquor, I had to severe some relationships with users and set healthier boundaries for myself with the others in my band. However, I am still working on triggers with a couple of family members, trust is something that has to be earned back, slowly, once it has been broken. Often, you can never really trust someone after they betray you. I found its best for me not to drink, to get in the state of mind to work on forgiveness and on allowing my inner child to heal and get over broken hearts and broken dreams. I've been working on myself and a new solo album. I will never get involved with abusers and users again. I am happy to say that 99% of the time I don't miss the alcohol, now..

Thanks for all your help and support. Your the best! Huggs, D.L

Write your own I Quit Alcohol Story Here:

____

____

The "I Quit" journal is a great additional therapy tool that gives you more space to journal your symptoms, thoughts and feelings during you sobriety journey. You can order it online.

I Quit !!!

The Quit or Die Book Journal

Quit Aid / First Aid/ Self-Work Book

A Guided Inward Journey On Your Path To Sobriety

Success Tips & Solutions For A Sober Lifestyle

Facing Problems Without Alcohol

Face problems instead of trying to drown them with alcohol, do it in the first place, rather than going through life having to continually ending relationships with a never-ending stream of abusive, dishonest people who continually take advantage of your goodness and kindness. Surround yourself with good people and you'll have less stress. Most importantly alcohol doesn't make your problems go away but it can keep you from having a problem solving mindset.

Everyone has problems at some point in their life, Alcohol is not a problem solver.

Counseling is always a good option whenever you are faced with problems that stump you. Learning what codependency and counter dependency is and learning how to break the cycle of emotional patterns and why we tend to get involved with same types of people and relationships is the only way to heal old emotional wounds that may drive you to drink your hurts away. You can't drink past hurts away. We can never have true happiness until we understand what drives our own destructive behaviors and do the self work to correct them. As long as you have a codependent personality, you will be the victim of a user/abuser predator because they can spot the people that they can victimize and target the cycle of use and abuse. it will be a repeating cycle in life if you don't work to heal your codependency roots and if they get away with betraying you once, they will do it again and again. Betrayal is an emotional wound that leads counter dependency and all can lead to addiction and alcoholism if not dealt with properly. Many drinkers tend to internalize their pain and numb it with Alcohol. Alcohol is an anesthetic. It is a trap. Don't fall into the Alcohol trap. Had I went through proper counseling my relapse in to codepency would have been less likely to occur and my alcohol abuse may have never happened. Therapy is not just for crazy people it can help us all.

People Make Mistakes

Forgiveness In Alcohol Recovery

To err is human, we all make mistakes. At some point we have to let go of past hurts and forgive so that we can heal and overcome addictions. Harboring resentment is toxic to our health and sobriety. Not forgiving only hurts yourself, the people that hurt us usually don't think about us afterwards and they move on with their lives, when we don't forgive them we allow ourself to be controlled by the emotional trauma of the ones who hurt us, don't give those idiots the power to further harm you. Forgive them and forget them. It's their loss. Most people will do what they can get away with instead of doing self work to correct character flaws, until they are caught or have a relationship crisis and have to make changes. Also, no one is perfect, everyone has something they can improve upon. Addiction is like an onion with many layers that have to be peeled back to get to the core emotional issue. It is always about the alcohol and the addictive nature of alcohol use, but it is the drug with the easiest access and that is why so many people self-medicate their pain with alcohol. Pain may be physical or linked to an emotional or behavior issue, abuse, neglect, addiction and various character flaws. There is always room for improvement. We all have the need to work on ourselves to grow and better ourselves. Counseling is always a good option, so is prayer and the bible says love one another and forgive one another. Forgiveness is the best form of love in any relationship. It takes a strong person to admit they are wrong and say they're sorry and an even stronger person to forgive.

> Albert Einstein once said, "The definition of insanity is doing the same thing over and over again, but expecting different results."

The time I had alcohol poisoning, I was on a sabbatical that went wrong, sometimes we can't run away from our problems rather work through them, together. Women are often expected to be seen and not heard. When we don't speak up that is when the predators will pounce. If someone has a predator mentality alcohol magnifies it and people end up hurt. In my relationship crisis, we took a sabbatical from each other, we each did our shadow work on our own and after four months apart, we took actions to correct the damage and settle disputes and debts to each other. In that time we gave up our addictions and held each other accountable. It helps to have an accountability partner. We talked through our differences, discussed each others expectations from the relationship and worked through our differences. We set new rules of respect and healthier boundaries, cleaned up use issues, made a commitment to support each other in recovery and decided to give our relationship a 2nd chance. Instead of running away, some problems can be worked on and resolved as friends. It was worth a second chance. Still, repeating the same mistake over with alcohol is a slip or a relapse. Some live through it, some don't.

"To err is human, to forgive divine" Alexander Pope

Alcohol Relapse Problems Resulting in Deaths

Relapse rates for alcohol fall within the 40-60 % range, so people often need support group, friends or hobbies to keep themselves happy and busy. If drinkers get bored they can relapse to the use of alcohol, even though it leads to problems. Alcoholism withdrawal, if mishandled, can result in death.The alcoholism relapse process may be the result of a progressive series of problems. My daughters dad had stopped drinking and was in a relationship that he was really into, it just didn't work out. He had an argument and was going through a breakup with his girlfriend and was unhappy about it and wanted to talk to her and try to work things out. He self-medicated his pain with alcohol and the night didn't go well, within days of a relapse and through a series of unfortunate events, he died. Alcohol was a factor. It is horrible to see anyone die that way.

Stress + Alcohol = Death

Stress is a killer and when we use alcohol to cope with stress and other problems it creates additional problems and makes all problems worse, not better. I had many years of healthy living and incredible educational and career successes. I had many fun and exciting adventures around the world, then there came a season of sadness in my life and I wasn't prepared. I had the image of going through life popping champagne corks when tragedies struck our family and within one year, my mom died, my daughters dad died, I almost died my family was bickering with me over my mom's end of life care, my celebrity business partner was taking our ideas and monetizing on them without me. My friend who promised to help my daughter further her career, wasn't keeping his promise, then his dad died and we all felt let down in life. I had a lot of expenses and financial stress, plus I was coming out of a long bout of counter dependency and having my first serious relationship in years turn into a catastrophe which put me under great stress. I was traumatized and I had my own near death experience due to high stress and poor stress management and self medicating with wine behind the scene. My friend Sonya and I use to get together and "wine" on each others shoulder about life's problems, but then we both quit "wine-ing" and most all our problems resolved within a year.

Alcohol Procrastinates Finding Solutions To Problems

Many people self-medicate their stress with alcohol and for me, wine was not the solution. In fact, it can kill you, just as it did my ex-husband, sadly, one fatal night via a mishandled alcohol overdose and a few days later I attended his funeral. My daughters father died of alcohol poisoning from having a blood alcohol level of over .385 and he did not have access to lifesaving emergency medical care. I saw how the death of my daughter's father broke the hearts of her, his mom and our family. All of these things happening at once, is when I chose to quit drinking wine, too. Hopefully, by my sharing my own horrible experience, you won't have to have a near death experience before you make the choice to quit, too.

Cracking Open A Can Of Whoop-Ass - Time To Quit

Eventually, alcohol will let you down and eventually you will see the negative effects outweigh the temporary feel good. You will wake up one day with your head pounding, sick with nausea from the worse hangover you ever had, shaking feeling like your nerves are shot and realize you wasted a lot of time and money on alcohol for nothing, really.The point is, life has its ups and downs, high's and low's, triumphs and setbacks, losses and failures but if you quit alcohol, you win. Life will always bring you joys and disappointments, that is just life. Life is so much richer and joyful without alcohol. Alcohol does not make any of life's experiences any better, statistically, and it's not the solution to your pain or problems. Alcohol is a temporary fix that distracts you and waste a lot of your time and money. The next day, you wake up in a fog trying to remember what you missed and your still stuck with the same problems and plus you have a headache and your hungover, to boot. Life is a tough enough struggle, without having your ass kicked by a bottle of booze. Quit wasting time in the pursuit of alcohol. Quit wasting your money on something that is destroying you and your health. Quit paying alcohol to kick your ass and keep you knocked off track in life. Just remember, the next time you crack open a cold one your opening up a can of whoop-ass on yourself. Quit alcohol and your life will get better in many ways.

How I Quit

There are a ton of methods for quitting alcohol. One good rule of thumb is, don't take advice from somebody you wouldn't switch lives with. Many people swap one addiction for another. I took time out to work through my emotional pain. Sometimes in life, we must do the thing we've been told not to, to get well. All of our lives we are taught to never be a quitter. At some point, the people who drink will make the choice to become a quitter. This is probably one of the only instances in life where your family will be glad that you became a quitter. Being a quitter is a great thing. Hopefully, you won't wait as long as I did to become a quitter, too. You see, I did have a few close calls before I decided that I never wanted to drink again. After our family experienced a death by alcohol, I was certain at that point, I would quit. I became soberingly aware of how alcohol use can end a person's life, and often when it does it is by a horrible death. I made up my mind I was quitting before I died from something related to alcohol, too. I research and found some of the natural substances listed in this book that have helped myself and many others relieve symptoms of addiction withdrawal. I read up on all the statistics regarding the negative effects of alcohol. I made a decision that I was not going to be just another statistic or one of the people who will die from alcohol. I decided to take control of my life back from alcohol. This book reveals how I did it. This is the approach that worked for me. There is no one-size-fits-all solution. There are many rehab options available. Hopefully, you find what works best for you.

Substance Abuse Is Less Likely When A Person Is In Good Emotional & Mental Health

Turning Negatives Into Positives

Life is beautiful, live each day like it's your last. Once upon a time, I had an overload of responsibilities, which was a recipe for misery. A person can only do so much, do not overload your life with burdens overload it with joy. You can't please, everyone, do your best but don't kill yourself trying. Dream big, but know that not all dreams come true. Life is full of disappointments, but can be filled with victories. When all else fails, there's always plan Z. People will let you down but it is worse to let yourself down. The higher you go, the further you fall. When life knocks you down, pick yourself up and try again. Heart's get broken but keep your heart open and love will mend it. Fill your heart with love and there will be no room for sorrow. Let your love light shine on the world. When someone betrays you, don't grow bitter, grow better. Alcohol may initially make you feel happy but eventually it betrays you. Noone has the power to drive you crazy unless you give them the keys. You have the power to take control of your life back, before alcohol destroys you. Nothing and no one has the power to ruin your life unless you give your power away to them.

Love That's Dead Alcohol Attraction

After your break-up with alcohol, one day you'll walk past the alcohol isle and say to yourself, glad I don't want that anymore. You may even be repulsed by the sight of the alcohol isle. For some or you, seeing alcohol may feel kind of like seeing an old lover that you wish it would have worked out with, but it didn't and you know it was best for you that you walked away because to have stayed in the relationship with alcohol you would have had a tragic ending. You are smarter, stronger and better because you moved beyond Alcohol. You no longer feel an intense attraction and just like a love-affair that has has ended you put it in the past and move on. You can still have mocktails and be able to easily put alcohol behind you, for the healthier version, too.

Healthy Relationships In Sobriety

Love is the drug we are all looking for. Our subconscious mind will keep bringing the same relationship issues up, in different relationships, until we do our shadow work and heal our wounded inner child. Same shit different relationship. The primary defining feature of a healthy autonomy is first that the autonomy motive is an "approach mindset," meaning that the individual desires to be self-reliant because they want to recognize their full potential as an individual, but one who is simultaneously and securely can interconnected with others forming lasting, loving relationships. Second, healthy autonomous individuals can regularly form effective, meaningful, intimate long term relations with others. That is, they can share, be vulnerable, and are comfortable relying on others when it is reasonable to do so.

To summarize what we've discovered together, alcohol is very damaging to your health, it numbs you and stunts your emotional growth, it damages your brain, heart, kidneys and your liver. It pickles you slowly over time. Alcohol can cause so much stress on your heart that it can cause a heart attack. Remember, love is the drug we are all looking for.

Divorcing Your Alcoholic Self

The maintenance of good emotional and mental health is important in the prevention of Alcohol abuse. In many drinkers, like myself, my emotionally wounded and battered "self" was the drinker. I had to do my emotional work. My shadow self was a drinker and I had to shed the shadow to step back into the person I really am. Alcohol changes personalities. Part of being in denial, is admitting that you suffer with alcohol related problems because we have to identify our emotional triggers, they are what sabotage our sobriety. Look deeply into yourself and your past, you will find the clues to the reasons you turned to alcohol to comfort something inside. I had emotional problems since I was 10 years old when my dad got killed and my mom was in survival mode, she had to be strong to be a single working mom supporting two children on her own. She didn't have the energy to deal with my emotions, and they were strong, I remember she told me to stop throwing a fit and crying over my dad that he was gone to heaven and was in a better place. I was the type of child that if he was in a better place, I wanted to go there too. I wanted to see him, right now. Mom said you cant you have to die before you see him again, so I said I wanted to kill myself to go see daddy, right now. I remember feeling like my dad and I had a lot of unfinished business, he kind of left without saying goodbye to me, properly. I missed him terribly and by age 12 I was angry at him for leaving me in this world all alone without a father. I had a devastating childhood wounding for which I did not receive proper grief counseling. From that wounding, my shadow-self was born. Poorly managed emotional and mental health care can lead to alcohol abuse, alcoholism and other diseases related to addiction. For years, I didn't know why I had the emotional blueprint for love in relationships or why I had a propensity to self-medicate with alcohol. The people I chose to keep company with drank, so I drank. When I figured out why and became aware of the reasons driving my behavior, it was easy to quit drinking. Looking back I can see that we all had similar emotional issues and poor coping mechanisms. Misery loves company. Alcohol is a form of self harm and punishment. After I healed the wounded inner child and gave myself unconditional love, I divorced my adult alcohol abusing self and I got the real me back. If you try, you can quit, too.

Getting The Real You, Back

So many people lose everything due to their use of alcohol that became destructive. The worst thing you can lose is yourself. If you are reading this book, it means, it's not too late for you to quit, things have not gone too far, yet. Before I quit I was headed toward trouble When I quit alcohol, I got my energy back, I got my motivation back, I got my positive nature back. Now the real me is back. The real me is drug and alcohol free. The real me is full of energy, love and life. Life is a struggle for most of us without the weight of carrying an extra ball and chain in the metaphorical form of an alcohol addiction weighing you down and sedating you. You can get your energy, motivation and joy back, too, by breaking the chains of addiction and quitting alcohol. Life is too short to waste it in a drunken stupor, heal your emotional wounds, stop picking your emotional wounds and allow the scabs to heal, the scars will also heal with time after you do your emotional work.

Emotional Wounds

Unlike physical wounds that you can see cuts, bruises, emotional wounds are felt inside. We have no emergency medical system to render emotional first aid, so we have to learn to manage these wounds sometimes with the help of professional counselors and support groups and we have to do our homework by ourselves. Therapy is not just for victimized people it can help us all. Picking open old painful emotional wounds is like picking open a scab and making a wound bleed again. It is called ruminating. Rumination is one of the similarities between anxiety and depression. Ruminating is simply repetitively going over an emotional injury or painful thought or problem without completion, resolve or healing. It is an obsessive painful thought. When people are hurt and depressed, the themes of rumination are typically about being inadequate or because someone important to you didn't make you feel important or valued, or maybe someone deliberately hurt you and it made you feel worthless or the other person made you feel your need were unimportant, maybe they took advantage of you. No one has the power to make you feel anything unless you give them the power. Meanwhile, that person had issues and maybe they took you for granted and maybe you can have a constructive conversation to work through problems in a healthy manner so that both of your needs and expectations are met. Regardless, of what someone else says or does, you are as valuable as you see your own self. Work on bettering your own sense of value and self worth. Put yourself and your needs first. Take care of yourself. Don't harm yourself with alcohol. If you have a compulsion that you can't seem to overcome on your own, seek help from a professional. If you can't do it alone, often, a counselor can help.

Journaling Your Way Through Sobriety

Keeping a sobriety journal is a way of getting in touch with your thoughts feelings and emotions and for keeping track of your sobriety birthday. Get a journal every year and keep track of your success and milestones.

Hypnosis

Is a behavior modification technique, that best works to help bring self-awareness regarding bad habits, fears and phobias. Hypnosis puts you in a hyper suggestible state of hyper-awareness. In the state of hypnosis, a person may access a deeper realms of their subconscious mind than in a usual state of awareness. Hypnosis is beneficial by helping to improve your understanding of how your subconscious mind drives your behaviors. In other words, hypnotic relaxation techniques can help you access your subconscious mind and uncover hidden root causes of alcohol use and addiction. For those struggling with alcohol abuse, hypnotherapy may help you understand why and how your drinking behaviors are driven. Additionally, it may help you learn and understand how to implement healthier behaviors in place of old or destructive behaviors. It is a good therapy for calming the mind and learning alternative relaxation techniques rather than using alcohol to chemically induce a fake or temporary relaxed state. Also, it may help with repressed emotions that result from abuse. Furthermore, during a professional hypnosis session, a person can examine their life more deeply to pinpoint behaviors that need change in order to cope with healthier methods of stress management and to view alcohol in a more realistic way. Many people suffering from alcohol abuse find it hard to admit that they have a substance abuse problem, denial is a major culprit in alcohol abuse and is the primary reason alcohol abuse goes untreated for years. Hypnosis compliments other rehab treatment methods and may be a viable part of a successful alcohol treatment plan. For most individuals hypno-therapy may help improve alcohol cessation outcomes for a lifetime of sobriety success.

The Keys To Sobriety

Part of the key to sobriety is understanding why withdrawal happens and allowing your body the time it needs to recovery. When you quit alcohol, there will be a period of Anhedonia, it is a condition in which the capacity of experiencing pleasure is totally or partially lost. Knowing how to support your mind and body with the extra care it needs to repair the physical damage and offset the uncomfortable feelings and symptoms of withdrawal until you can be comfortable in sobriety. Anhedonia has been found to be a frequent feature in alcoholics and other addicted patients during acute and chronic withdrawal stages. Utilizing an integrative sobriety support system as part of your getting sober strategy and staying sober lifelong lifestyle plan. You need to be aware and harness the proper tools and weapons to help you win your battle, physically and mentally to regain your strength in sobriety. It is important to eat a balanced healthy diet with additional nutritional support for the neurotransmitter system so it has adequate building blocks to aid in the recovery process. Anhedonia makes you feel like you've lost your sense of pleasure and makes you feel like something is wrong or not right in your body. It can be worrisome, as this is a state where many have self-harming thoughts and requires professional help if it gets to that point. Anhedonia refers to both a mental state and physical symptoms and a personality trait, it feels like a dark cloud hovering over you, it may feel impossible to smile, you may feel sad, it is a feeling of loss each quitter has to divorce themself from. Alcohol has a dopaminergic mesolimbic and mesocortical reward circuit. Anhedonia frequently occurs in mood disorders and as a negative symptom in substance use disorders due to several factors including brain chemistry imbalance due to alcohol dependence.

Anhedonia is a factor not only in the alcohol dependent but also amphetamine, cocaine and cannabis abusers can also experience it, as well. In all those with a substance dependence disorder, there is a significant correlation between being in the state of anhedonia and craving intensity, withdrawal, psychosocial and altered personality characteristics. Therefore treating anhedonia in alcohol-detox subjects and can be critical in terms of relapse prevention, given its strong relationship with craving.

Additionally, doing physical therapies for physical pain and doing emotional work and shadow work to resolve and quit ruminating old emotional wounds. I am not talking about putting on a fake smile and pretending like everything's alright, when it's not. I am talking about getting real with yourself and sometimes that requires getting down into the deepest darkest part of your shadow self, facing emotions and working through them and flooding the darkness with truth, love and light. Facing your fears and problems and resolving them. Learning how to love every part of yourself, especially the parts of yourself that you secretly dislike. Using the energy that you may be wasting on alcohol or being angry and feeling victimized and channeling it to improve your situation, to get better, not bitter. Everyone has an inner child and everyone has a shadow self. Help your inner child heal. Get in touch with it. To thy own self, be true.

You can finally be free of the heavy burden of carrying old emotional wounds that drive you to make impulsive decisions and make wiser decisions about your drinking, your life and your health so you can quit numbing the pain or swallowing emotions with alcohol.

You still have time. The bible teaches us that of all things there are three things that last forever, and they are faith, hope and love and it says that the greatest of them all is love. Let past hurts go, allow your heartbreaks to heal. Therefore, part of healing is forgiving. Forgive yourself for causing self harm by drinking, and forgive those that have hurt you or caused you pain or harm. Finally, surround yourself with self-love, forgiveness, understanding, acceptance and sobriety. The bible also says, love one another and forgive one another. That doesn't mean you have to stay miserable with someone who abuses you and continually disrespects you or causes you ANY harm. You still have to weed those types of people out of your life and put them in the past so you can move on to a better future.

Even if you don't want to get into the scriptures, know that the past is the past, and find a way to be at peace in letting it go. We do not live in the past nor do we live in the future. We live in the present. This second, right now, this is the only moment in time that you have control of. Look at your watch. You can decide how you react in each moment. Each second you will make the decision not to drink in every passing second. Wear a watch or program it into an app on your computer or phone, start counting the seconds of your sobriety.

Our lives are experienced in seconds. We make choices that create our future, a new path in life begins now and in each and every second. Your life passes by each second, and seconds turn into minutes, and minutes turn to hours and hours turned to days and days turned into weeks and weeks turn to months and months turn to years, and years. There is no point in worrying about the future. The key to being successful in sobriety comes in the decision you make not to drink alcohol each and every second in present time, for the rest of your life. It is a choice. You have total and willful control over that choice once you remove all the reasons to drink then all you have left are the reasons not to drink and there are a million reasons in this book why to quit drinking. Love is the drug we all need. Love yourself, don't abuse yourself with alcohol.

I hope you make the choice to quit, too. I hope I have at least helped you become more aware and perhaps even utterly disgusted by the damaging effects of alcohol and that once you realize that you have been sold a lie by alcohol advertisers that it makes you angry enough to quit. I hope this story help motivate you to quit an over-drinking habit. Those of us who survive alcoholism, it is through self-work that makes us stronger. Quitting isn't easy but it shows that you have power and control over your own life and it is a sign of amazing strength. Think of the one thing you do best in life and apply the skills of how you do that thing, to your sobriety and you will be successful.

Drinking Alcohol is not cool, it doesn't make you more sexy or attractive or smarter, in fact, it makes you the opposite! Alcohol is not glamorous nor is it a symbol of success. The truth is Alcoholism is an addictive drug that ruins lives. Alcohol ruins families, Alcohol ruins jobs. Alcohol damages your brain, mind and body. Alcohol robs you of your good health, your beauty and your money. Alcohol can cause you legal problems, DUI's and causes accidents. Alcohol is can be as deadly as a bullet. Alcohol kills. You can regain control of your life and take your power back. It is time to break up your relationship with alcohol. Kick the habit, kick alcohol out of your life. Take your power back. Restore your joy, hope and motivation. All you have to do is kick alcohol out of your life and start living again. Take control, you have the power to quit drinking before it kills you. In life, none of us are guaranteed another day and none of us will make it out of here alive but we can potentially, have a better chance to live longer, if we quit drinking.

Encouraging Words From Our Presidents

I give you the same advice that our current president, Donald Trump, personally gave to me: "Develop Stick-To-It-Tiveness and you will be successful". Actually, he was giving me business advice and what he said was, "Do what you love and love what you do and develop stick-to-it-tiveness and you will be successful in all you do". This can be applied to your sobriety success, as well and is so important to all of us, especially those recovering from alcohol and addiction to develop stick-to-it-tiveness. Additionally, in the spirit of our past president Obama, who always encouraged the American people with his slogan; Yes, we can!!! He was so positively motivating for us with those three words and it is still a reminder to us all today to keep a positive attitude, do the work and believe that we shall overcome the problems we face and again their words can apply to the alcoholism epidemic, too. Yes, we can find a solution for all obstacles along the path to sobriety. It may not be easy to give up alcohol but by understanding why it is a struggle and arming yourself with a stick-to-it attitude and the tools and methods for success described herein can help ease the struggle and the pain of withdrawal so that it will be easier for you to achieve success in sobriety.

In 1978, the World Health Organisation, defined Anhedonia as a widespread depressed mood of gloom and wretchedness with some degree of anxiety. This describes the feelings of despair felt during alcohol rehab and addiction recovery. It is a very uncomfortable stage for both mind and body, but, one of the best things you can do to feel better, in the future. Start doing the things you really love to do that give you a great sense of pleasure. Before you spent all that time getting boozed up or high, you likely had hobbies, things you did that you really use to enjoy doing before you became an addict. Start doing those hobbies again as soon as possible. Exercise is a must as it stimulates all the feel good hormones in the body and mind. If you use to golf or go boating, jet skiing, fishing, bowling, playing ball or any hobby that truly made you feel happy, do it. Do the things you use to love, again. Every little thing you can do to offset the feeling of anhedonia, the better and the more likely you will be able to stay sober and live in sobriety for a lifetime.

You Can Quit - Yes You Can!

You can quit, too. There are so many options to be a success in your sobriety. There are many helpful natural foods, supplements and counseling programs available. I used the information in this book and had some therapies that helped me feel better. It worked for me and for many people I know, but every person is different and each person may need to tweak this self-care approach, and a few may even need a different therapeutic approach while some others may need to take an inpatient rehab approach.

I successfully Quit wine and I'm doing great by utilizing the tips within this book. The best thing is my joy, energy and motivation are back. I didn't realize how sedated wine made me feel. After I quit, my health and life has improved dramatically for the better in many ways and yours can, too.

Remember, the facts, be strong, god bless you and good luck to you. Now, you have two choices, hopefully, you will make the healthy choice before alcohol destroys your life or kills you. What will you decide to do, "Quit or Die"?

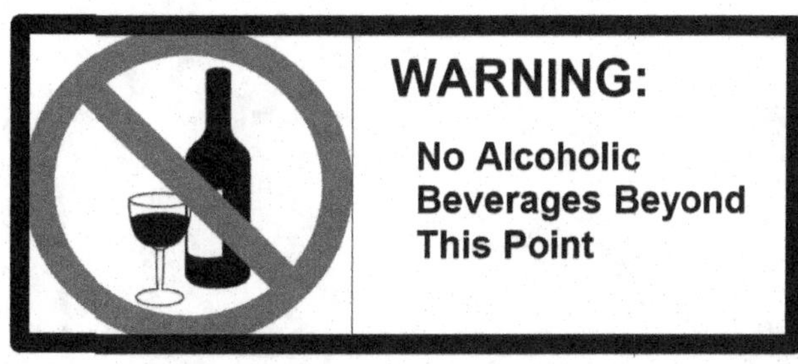

Victory Is Yours!

Disclaimers

If you you or your family members are suffering or struggling with alcoholism, do not be afraid to seek help. You do not have to face this alone, there are many health professionals and rehab facilities options available. Additionally, The fact sheets by the FDA and the Office of Dietary Supplements provides information that should not take the place of medical advice. We encourage you to talk to your healthcare providers (doctor, addiction counselor, registered dietitian, pharmacist, etc.) about your interest in, questions about, or use of dietary supplements and what may be best for your overall health. Any mention in this publication of a specific product or service, or recommendation from an organization or professional society, does not represent an endorsement by the author of that product, service, or as expert advice. As always, please seek the advice of your physician before starting any new health plan. Additionally, seek out community public health programs as approved by government agencies that provide information on alcohol, tobacco and drug awareness as well as prescription and over the counter medications, consumer drug information, and reports and publications.

References

CDC - Center For Disease Control

NIH - National Institutes of Health

FDA- Food and Drug Administration

Harvard Medical Research

National Suicide Prevention Lifeline 1-800-273-8255

World Health Organization WHO.org

Drugabuse.com

Wikipedia - Alcohol statistics

National Organization on Fetal Alcohol Syndrome

Foundation for Advancing Alcohol Responsibility

New England Journal Of Medicine

Responsibility.org

Debbieford.com

Bettyfordclinic.com

National Association Of Addiction Treatment Providers.

Whitehouse.archives.gov

Monarch Shores Rehabilitation

Addiction Centers of America

American Addiction Centers

Evergreen Drug Rehab Centers

Alcohol.org

U.S. National Library of Medicine

National Institutes of Health.

http: www.nlm.nih.gov medlineplus druginformation.html

Center for Drug Evaluation and Research: http: www.fda.gov cder

http: www.fda.gov drugs resources for you

National Institute on Alcohol Abuse and Alcoholism

http: www.niaaa.nih.gov

Phone number: 301–443–3860

Main FDA for general inquiries:

Free informational materials on alcohol use, alcohol abuse, and alcoholism.

Drug Reaction: Medwatch: 1–800–FDA–1088

1–888–INFO–FDA (1–888–463–6332)

Clinical Studies References

Depression Research and Treatment Luigi Grillo, Volume 2016, Article ID 1598130

Yale J Biol Med. 2015 Sep; 88(3): 325–332. Published online 2015 Sep 3. PMCID: PMC4553654 PMID: 26339217 Focus: Addiction

Geriatric Orthopedic Surgery & Rehabilitation 2010 Sep; 1(1): 6–14.

doi: 10.1177/2151458510378105 PMCID: PMC3597289PMID: 23569656

MILLER, B.A.; MAGUIN, E.; AND DOWNS, W.R. Alcohol, drugs, and violence in children's lives. In: Galanter, M., ed. *Recent Developments in Alcoholism: Volume 13. Alcoholism and Violence.* New York: Plenum Press, 1997. pp. 357-385.

SCHUCK, A.M., AND WIDOM, C.S. Childhood victimization and alcohol symptoms in females: An examination of causality and hypothesized mediators. *Child Abuse & Neglect*, in press.

WIDOM, C.S. Child abuse, neglect, and witnessing violence. In: Stoff, D.; Breiling, J.; and Maser, J., eds. *Handbook of Antisocial Behavior.* New York: Wiley, 1997. pp. 159-179.

WIDOM, C.S. Post traumatic stress disorder in abused and neglected children grown up. *American Journal of Psychiatry* 156:1223-1229, 1999.

WIDOM, C.S.; IRELAND, T.; AND GLYNN, P.J. Alcohol abuse in abuse and neglected children followed-up: Are they at increased risk? *Journal of Studies on Alcohol* 56(2):207-217, 1995.

Glossary

ALCOHOLISM- an addiction to alcohol

BINGE DRINKING: According to the government, binge drinking is defined as the consumption of five or more (for males) and four or more (for females) drinks in a row in about two hours at least once in the past two weeks. The NIAAA defines binge drinking as a pattern of drinking alcohol that brings the BAC level to .08 or above.

HEAVY ALCOHOL USE: According to the government, heavy alcohol use is defined as five or more drinks on the same occasion on 5 or more days in the past 30 days.

UNDERAGE DRINKING: Underage drinking refers to the consumption of beverage alcohol, defined as a can or bottle of beer, a glass of wine or a wine cooler, a shot of distilled spirits, or a mixed drink with distilled spirits in it, by persons 20 years of age and younger.

Since 1988, all 50 states and the District of Columbia have laws that make it illegal for anyone under the age of 21 to purchase or publicly possess beverage alcohol. While each state's law varies and may contain exceptions (e.g., religious ceremonies) it is generally considered illegal for anyone under 21 to consume alcohol.

Drunk Driving Glossary

ALCOHOL-IMPAIRED DRIVING FATALITY: Drivers in all 50 states and D.C. are considered to be alcohol-impaired if their blood alcohol concentration (BAC) is .08 grams per deciliter (g/dL) or higher. Any fatality occurring in a crash that involves at least one driver or motorcycle operator with a BAC of .08 percent or higher is considered to be an alcohol-impaired fatality.

ALCOHOL-INVOLVED TRAFFIC FATALITY: A traffic fatality is considered alcohol-related if either the driver or anyone else involved in the police reported crash other than a passenger (e.g., a pedestrian or bicyclist) has alcohol in their bloodstream (a BAC level of .01 percent or more).

For example, if a pedestrian with a BAC of .01 percent steps off the curb in front of a sober driver and is killed by that driver, the fatality is included in alcohol-related traffic statistics. If a driver who has been drinking hits a car with two sober people in it and kills both, those two fatalities are considered alcohol-involved. In producing national and state statistics, NHTSA estimates the extent of alcohol involvement when alcohol test results are unknown.

ASSESSMENT: Depending on the discipline, the term "assessment" can refer to a variety of methods used to determine the nature of a problem and course of action needed to correct the problem. In general, criminal justice assessment tools fall into three basic categories: screening instruments, comprehensive risk/needs assessments, and specialized tools.

SCREENING INSTRUMENTS: Are generally quick and easy to use and focus more on static risk factors, such as a person's criminal history or potential substance use concerns. Screening tools can be useful in making quick determinations about in-or-out decisions (e.g., who should be detained, who should be released on their own recognizance), in helping to classify offenders into low, moderate or high risk categories or whether a more thorough substance abuse or mental health assessment should be conducted. However, their usefulness is somewhat limited since they do not help the practitioner identify an offender's criminogenic factors or the unique issues they have related to substance abuse or mental health.

COMPREHENSIVE RISK/NEEDS ASSESSMENT: Cover all major risk and needs factors (both static and dynamic) and help ascertain levels of risk and/or need that are correlated with outcome measures like recidivism. These assessments can also be useful in re-assessment to determine if needs changed after interventions have been introduced. The results from these assessments should be used to facilitate the development of case plans that can be aimed at addressing a full range of factors.

SPECIALIZED TOOLS: Specialized tools include things like alcohol and drug assessments. Typically, these types of assessments are the ones in which judges refer offenders to other professionals for. The key is that when referrals are made and these types of assessments are done, that the results be provided to and considered by judges so they can be used in the formulation of a supervision plan.

BINGE DRINKING: According to the National Institute on Alcohol Abuse and Alcoholism (NIAAA), binge drinking is defined as occasions of heavy drinking measured by the consumption of five or more (for males) and four or more (for females) drinks in a row at least once in the past two weeks.

BLOOD ALCOHOL CONCENTRATION: BAC is measured in grams of alcohol per 100 milliliters of blood. A BAC of .01 percent indicates .01 grams of alcohol per 100 milliliters of blood. By July 2004, all 50 states and the District of Columbia have passed legislation establishing that a driver with a BAC of .08 percent is considered legally intoxicated. Additionally, 42 states and the District of Columbia have laws and penalties for those who drive with elevated or "high" BAC levels.

COMMUNITY CORRECTIONS: A component of the criminal justice system which offers programs and services in the community and/or viable alternatives to incarceration for individuals at various stages of the criminal justice process. Community corrections may include bail/bond programs; behavior change strategies; restitution, fines and fees collection; probation and parole supervision; electronic monitoring; community service; and day reporting centers.

COMMUNITY SUPERVISION: Refers to the conditional release and supervision of defendants/offenders in a community setting. A conditional release of a defendant/offender to community supervision can occur at varying times in the criminal justice process, including pre- trialpretrial, pre-sentence, and post-sentence. Additionally, the availability of various community corrections supervision strategies vary by jurisdiction as resources vary.

DIVERSION PROGRAMS: A criminal justice program run by either a police department, court, a district attorney's office, probation department or outside agency designed to afford offenders the opportunity to avoid criminal charges and a criminal record by completing various requirements dictated by the program (e.g. drug treatment, counseling, community service). Successful completion of all requirements could result in dismissal or reduction of charges; whereas, non-completion of requirements could result in more serious action being taken by the court.

HARDCORE DRUNK DRIVERS: Hardcore drunk drivers are those who drive with a high BAC of .15 percent or above, or who drive repeatedly with a .08 percent or greater BAC, as demonstrated by having more than one impaired driving arrest, and are highly resistant to changing their behavior despite previous sanctions, treatment, or education.

HEAVY ALCOHOL USE: Five or more drinks on the same occasion on five or more days in the past 30 days.

IMPAIRED DRIVING: The state in which a driver who operates a motor vehicle is drunk (BAC=.08+), drugged, distracted and/or drowsy while driving.

INTENSIVE SUPERVISION PROGRAMS (ISP): These programs are often viewed as an alternative to incarceration. Persons sentenced to ISP are typically those who, in the absence of intensive supervision, would have been sentenced to imprisonment.

No two jurisdictions operate intensive supervision in exactly the same way. However, one characteristic of all ISPs is that they provide for very strict terms of probation or parole. This increased level of control is usually achieved through reduced caseloads, increased number of contacts, and a range of required activities that can include treatment services, victim restitution, community service, employment, random urine and alcohol testing, electronic monitoring, and payment of a supervision fee.

PAROLE: Any form of release of an offender from an institution (jail, prison) to the community by a releasing authority (parole board) prior to the expiration of an imposed sentence. Upon release, the offender may be subject to an array of supervision terms and conditions.

PROBATION: A sentencing option whereby an offender who has been found guilty of a crime is permitted to remain in the community under court supervision. Typically, the court will impose conditions of supervision, such as paying a fine, completing community service activities, participating in drug and/or mental health treatment, and education/employment requirements, which will be monitored by a probation officer. Failure to comply with the imposed terms could result in the offender being incarcerated to finish out the imposed sentence.

REPEAT OFFENDERS: The NHTSA/FARS data records prior driving records (convictions only, not violations) for driving while intoxicated events occurring within three years of the date of the crash. The same driver can have one or more of these convictions during this three year period. Drivers who have a prior conviction in this three year period are reported as repeat offenders.

RESPONSIVITY: Refers to the practice of considering individual characteristics (such as learning style, culture, gender, motivation level) when assigning individuals to community supervision and treatment programs.

STANDARD DRINK OF ALCOHOL: According to the Dietary Guidelines for Americans, the federal government's official nutrition policy defines a standard drink of alcohol as 1.5 ounces of 80-proof distilled spirits, 12 ounces of regular beer or 5 ounces of wine.

STAGGERED SENTENCING: A court-ordered sentence, most notably used with DWI offenders, which mixes periods of incarceration with periods of community supervision. The court places an offender on probation for a specified time period, and orders a period of incarceration to be served in two or more installments occurring during the probation period. These installments are spaced several months to one year apart. The offender must serve the first incarceration segment immediately or soon after the sentencing date, and is advised by the court of the dates on which the offender must begin serving subsequent incarceration segments.

If the offender attains goals during the periods of community supervision (such as treatment goals, sobriety goals, compliance goals) then the offender can submit a motion to the sentencing judge to waive the next installment of incarceration. This sentencing model allows the offender to influence their sentencing outcomes. (NHTSA, 2004).

UNDERAGE DRINKING: Since 1988, all 50 states and the District of Columbia have laws that make it illegal for anyone under the age of 21 to purchase or publicly possess alcoholic beverages. While each state's law varies and may contain exceptions (e.g., religious ceremonies) it is generally considered illegal for anyone under 21 to consume alcohol. Underage drinking refers to the consumption of beverage alcohol, defined as defined as a can or bottle of beer, a glass of wine or a wine cooler, a shot of distilled spirits, or a mixed drink with distilled spirits in it, by persons 20 years of age and younger.

WOMEN AND ALCOHOL: Women have less fluid in their bodies than men of the same weight, so there's less water to dilute alcohol. So with the same amount of alcohol, women will generally feel and experience the effects of alcohol more than men.

Product Resources

QuitAid

AidBrand.com http://www.aidbrand.com

Anti Aging Brand - http://www.antiagingbrand.com

CBD-Aid

Quit CBD (products from non-cannabis food sources)

AlcoTabs

AlcoEase

KudChews

Quitamine - Dietary Supplement

Essential Oils

Monoterpenes

Kombucha-tea

QuitAidTM- Effervecent Drink Tablets